Youth Ministries:
SEXUAL PURITY

by
Elnora Wilson

AuthorHouse™
1663 Liberty Drive, Suite 200
Bloomington, IN 47403
www.authorhouse.com
Phone: 1-800-839-8640

First published by AuthorHouse 5/16/2008

ISBN: 978-1-4343-3474-9 (sc)

Library of Congress Control Number: 2007907278

Printed in the United States of America
Bloomington, Indiana

This book is printed on acid-free paper.

This book is dedicated to Lamar, Chelsi, Candace,
and my late mother, Lurelia Smith

Preface

God discloses through his Word an incredible need for love, fellowship, liberty, and compassion in the body of Christ. Christians must come together to accomplish His purpose for our lives. Many of us go through life with no identity because we fail to make God a priority in our lives. Therefore, we live powerless lives and fall into many sins.

We say that we are empowered by the Lord...He is our fortress yet we often lose sight of where our help comes from. We try on our own to be free from bondages such as: fornication, intimidation, insecurity, being ashamed of Christ and others. Too often we overlook the fact that we are powerless without God.

We should be helping one another deal with disappointments, temptations, confusion, loneliness, and unite our efforts to help the feeble minded and be a witness to the unbelievers. The power of God lives in us to do the work of Christ as His ambassadors. When united, we become stronger and we can accomplish more work in the body of Christ.

Unfortunately, Satan causes confusion and division among Christians which results in an increase in abortions, divorces, fornication, adultery, homosexuality, lesbianism, and many other sins. Don't misunderstand my point, the body of Christ will never be destroyed, but division in the church causes confusion within the body. It's not enough to say that we are Christians but we must believe it within our hearts and demonstrate it in our lives.

When God inspired me to write this book, it was just an assignment, now it has become much more. After studying and hearing the word of God being taught by pastors, teachers, etc. so much has become clearer to me. For instance, many children want the truth and to be disciplined as long as it doesn't interfere with their schedule. They also know that fornication is wrong, but they rely on grace for forgiveness. We must take responsibility for our actions in order to make a difference.

I want this book to inspire children to think before they act. I would like for them to listen to the friend that encourages good things and not the associate who doesn't care about consequences. I pray that they will seek God on their level of understanding to increase spiritual growth and allow him to use them for His purpose.

The basic concept of this book is to encourage children to live by Christian morals. Encouraging them to…

Know who you are in Christ…that the world can't define you.

Know who you are…that you won't be talked into a sexual relationship.

Know who you are…that you won't be ashamed of Jesus Christ.

Know who you are…that you won't live in insecurity.

Know who you are…that you won't live in intimidation.

Know who you are…that you will walk boldly in the will of the Lord.

If children will take this book seriously it may possibly teach them to be wise when making choices and how to make sound decisions in secular matters, which is why I reiterated several points throughout this book to perhaps keep the focus on a spiritual perspective.

Acknowledgements:

For personal time spent to improve the text, grateful acknowledgement is extended to the following individuals:

General Editor
Dorothy Fancher
Charles Johnson

Graphic Editors
Sharon Vincent
Charsl McGhee

Contents

Introduction

(The Christian Walk in God's inspired word)

In the King James Version of The Holy Bible God's word tells us the following: *Ephesians 4:13-32 13Till we all come in the unity of the faith, and of the knowledge of the Son of God, unto a perfect man, unto the measure of the stature of the fullness of Christ: 14That we henceforth be no more children, tossed to and fro, and carried about with every wind of doctrine, by the sleight of men, and cunning craftiness, whereby they lie in wait to deceive; 15But speaking the truth in love, may grow up into him in all things, which is the head, even Christ: 16From whom the whole body fitly joined together and compacted by that which every joint supplieth, according to the effectual working in the measures of every part, maketh increase of the body unto the edifying of itself in love. 17This I say therefore, and testify in the Lord, that ye henceforth walk not as other Gentiles walk, in the vanity of their mind, 18Having the understanding darkened, being alienated from the life of God through the ignorance that is in them, because of the blindness of their* heart: *19Who being past feeling have given themselves over unto lasciviousness, to work all uncleanness with greediness. 20But ye have not so learned Christ; 21If so be that ye have heard him, and have been taught by him, as the truth is I Jesus: 22That ye put off concerning the former conversation the old man, which is corrupt according to the deceitful lusts; 23And be renewed in the spirit of your mind; 24And that ye put on the new man, which after God is created in righteousness and true holiness. 25Wherefore putting away lying, speak every man truth with his neighbour: for we are members one of another. 26Be ye angry, and sin not: let not the sun go down upon your wrath: 27Neither give place to the devil. 28Let him that stole steal no more: but rather let him labour, working with his hands the thing which is good, that he may have to give to him that needeth. 29Let no corrupt communication proceed out of your mouth, but that which is good to the use of edifying, that it may minister grace unto the hearers. 30And grieve not the holy Spirit of God, whereby ye are sealed unto the day of redemption. 31Let all bitterness, and wrath, and anger, and clamour, and evil speaking, be put away from you, with all malice: 32And be ye kind one to another, tenderhearted, forgiving one another, even as God for Christ's sake hath forgiven you.*

Self-worth

Teenagers live energetic, spontaneous lives for the most part, perhaps even daring for those who like to venture out on the adrenaline. Sometimes with very little thought of the outcome their will to be adventurous consume the thought process. The challenge of succeeding makes it even more exciting to proceed into the danger zone. Although there is no hesitation to become a part of the unknown, a part of them has to wonder what the next day will hold when all of the excitement quiets down. The possibilities are endless; unfortunately, many of them take the risk then hope for the best. The alternative would be considering who they are in Christ and remember that self-worth holds more value than popular, "teen happenings."

Self-Worth is the image resulting from an individual's conduct. What makes something or someone valuable? Value exists in everyone, but the extent of that value depends on the individual and how they view themselves. Webster's dictionary defines value as a quality that makes something more or less acceptable or useful.

What is your life worth? Is there a price that you would place on your life by taking unnecessary risks? Would you risk losing your self respect by stripping before others? Would you risk your life to engage in a sexual encounter? Would you risk losing a relationship for a one night stand? Examine yourself to determine the level of your self worth. One night or one moment can destroy an image that took years to define resulting in an extended number of years to redefine.

We can find ourselves in an addiction if we are not careful, but the acknowledgement of that addiction is called the turning point, not the dwelling place. What would it take for you to visualize the big picture of your life and not limit it to the view that's currently before you? Find your place of recovery and make that your starting point for spiritual growth. It does no good to know better, but remain in the very acts that are destroying you. Whether we realize it or not, someone is observing us and may want to be like us. What examples are we setting? Our choices are not always about "self."

The choices we make will determine our destiny as well as build our reputation and character. Our choices will also determine our eternal destination after life on earth is over. Some might say that life is simple, while others might say, "Life is complicated and full of uncertainties." The fact is life is our perception of the truth. But what is the truth? The truth is not what I believe, nor is it what the next person believes. Truth is an actual existence, which can't be tampered with, nor changed, neither can it be watered down and still maintain its abilities. Whether it is accepted or rejected, it always has been and it will always be. One can't hide from the truth, because it will always find you out.

Unlike people, truth can only serve its purpose and do the very thing that it is. Some people are discontented about many things in their lives. For example. At conception, God made us either male or female, but many have decided that God made a mistake and have consulted with physicians to change their sex. God created marriage for a man and a woman, but a number of individuals have chosen unnatural affections, and are engaging in same sex relationships. These behaviors complicate life. We have left the basics searching for something new. There is an end to all of this confusion and in the end when life for each of us is over we will be confronted with the truth. Jesus Christ is the source of all truth. This fact will make some happy to have chosen to live by it and will make others sad because they rejected it. As a result of rejecting Him, there are many physical diseases known as sexually transmitted diseases (STDs). If we stay in God's plan of resisting fornication, adultery, homosexuality, lesbianism, bi-sexuality, masturbation, oral & anal sexual methods, and other sexual sins, STDs could be avoided.

Sexually transmitted diseases are the results of our bad choices. The decision to abstain from sexual intercourse of any sort is wise and assuring. There is no other choice that guarantees safety from STDs. The secular world believes that the concept of proper condom usage will prevent STDs. This is not actual and certainly not a proven fact. Celibacy not only prevents STDs, but it also helps to maintain a moral lifestyle.

Let us also consider the positive impact on society by eliminating unwanted pregnancies. This will also do away with the sin of abortion. There are some health issues that make abortions necessary such as an ectopic pregnancy. The sin of abortion is killing an unborn child out of convenience. These issues and others are the results of leaving truth for self satisfaction.

Where do we draw the line? When do we make a stand for truth? Are we sold-out to worldliness? Infatuation mistaken for love, gift giving for self recognition, doing whatever it takes to get ahead; slander and deception are all actions that take away from ones character. How sad is it to pursue another's husband or wife, sneak around with teachers, plot to harm another individual out of jealousy, but fail to see the damage being done? Or how far are you willing to go only to reap the consequences of it later?

Good character is necessary for the proper development of a person. Physical growth is not the only requirement for development in an adult nor is physical maturity a good measure of a person's self worth. Although, some males believe that sexual relations with numerous females make them men, this is far from the truth. It takes away from their ability to define themselves as men. As young men, you can build on your masculinity to develop into godly men, the kind of men that godly women want. Females fall into this mindset as well, resulting in loss of character. Women who try to identify themselves through physical means such as: appearance, class, or financial statuses alone are likely victims of low self-esteem. Dressing nicely, keeping high standards in our appearance, and preference is good. We should never settle for less especially if the opportunity is there to achieve, accomplish, or have more. Attracting the opposite sex can be accomplished by being a person who lives by biblical standards and not necessarily by physical appearance. Physical attraction between male and female is only natural; however, sexual intimacy should be practiced within the guidelines of marriage.

Youth are sometimes lead by others to believe that sexual relations are fine as long as they are protected.

Some believe that this type of behavior is normal as long as it is under control. To teach such non-sense is a good example of bad leadership. Sex is a holy and sacred act when it is kept within the marriage relationship. *Hebrew 13:4 Marriage is honourable in all, and the bed undefiled: but whoremongers and adulterers God will judge (KJV).* Of course, this rule is often ignored and broken, which is why we have numerous individuals with STDs. Other problems that come from illicit sexual activity include: Overpopulation, economic issues, abortions, and single parent homes. These problems can be avoided by practicing abstinence and couples keeping sex within the marriage.

Sex has negatively impacted many industries such as: Entertainment, clothing, and music to name a few. Some people will not associate with you if you are not sexually involved. Unless a sexual affair is agreed upon, many have lost their jobs. Many companies have resorted to sexual contents in their commercials to sell their products.

We have to take a stand for morality, because the time is coming when we must put on immortality and be held accountable for the sins we've committed in our mortal bodies. *I Corinthians 15:53* reads, *For this corruptible must put on incorruption, and this mortal must put on immortality. (KJV)*

We live to have sex is the theory of some evolutionist. According to their belief, evolution has changed the physical appearance of the ape to the up right, face to face appearance of man. They have also concluded that it is the nature of man to want to reproduce; therefore, they feel manly when they act according to their nature. They believe that lust turns into love and love turns into lust. The Discovery Health Channel reported on the, "Anatomy of Sex," that four million years of evolution is the end product of two sex machines. Based on their theory, sex is an act with no guidelines just precautions due to STDs. Christians cannot live by those standards, because they do not acknowledge the creator. Evolutionists aren't concerned about godliness. They thrive to prove that God doesn't exist. And without God, there can be no sin and lifestyles such as homosexuality are just that…lifestyle. They also concluded that there is no life after death; neither does life begin at conception, which is why abortion is not an issue for many people.

Christians have to take a stand for Christ and remain faithful to that choice. We must be mindful of the information we receive and not allow worldly ideas to control our thoughts.

Maintaining abstinence is a willful act. We are human and are subject to physical and emotional sexual feelings. The biggest mistake we make is acting inappropriately on those emotions. Therefore, we must recognize and take control of these thoughts. When we control our thoughts, we control our physical and emotional urges. We must lose those thoughts immediately after they enter our minds to avoid acting on them.

We can keep our bodies pure if we keep our minds on God. It's a daily battle, which can be difficult or easy depending on our own willingness to resist temptation. Thinking beyond the body and placing emphasis on our spiritual being is part of the solution. Another method is encouraging one another and being self-motivated. It's easy to lose focus when we dwell on the lifestyle of others. It's easy to lose sight of things when we compare our own lives with someone who looks like he or she has it all together. For example, we may sometime become depressed when we see worldly couples living together, unmarried, have big houses, nice cars, and jobs that some only dream of having. You may experience low self-esteem by not accepting that lifestyle. Your friends constantly remind you of your decision and tell you about the person your ex is dating. It can be painful to hear about this great lifestyle that could have been yours. How do you deal with it? Or how do you get past the negativity of your friends for making the right choice?

For starters, you can think on the greater reward you will receive after this temporary life is over. Choices that benefit your eternal being is better than those which only benefits your physical being. Decisions that benefit both this world and the one to come are the best choices.

There are many sins, but fornication is a sin against the body. *I Corinthians 6:18* says, *Flee fornication. Every sin that a man doeth is without the body; but he that committeth fornication sinneth against his own body. (KJV)* Think of it this way; don't make yourself used goods to possibly become contaminated. As a result of sexual sin, STDs are spreading like wildfire, unfortunately, some of these diseases kill. Some people feel that they won't contract a sexually transmitted disease. The sad thing is, when the disease is transmitted it can't be undone. How valuable is your life? If an individual is willing to live with you without marriage, it is a simple way of saying, "I'll make you my live-in sex partner, but you are not worthy to have all of me." A portion of the check book and sex is what he or she is willing to give, which means that this person is free to do whatever is pleasing since there is no commitment.

Many of us can only see the here and now. Often times, we fail to consider the long-term effects of our decisions. Fun, fun, and more fun dominates the lives of many people. Sex is more of a hobby or maybe a sport for some and even a contest for others. We have to abandon this mindset. Unknowingly, it's going to destroy those who fail to cease sexual sins or any sin for that matter. *Romans 6:23 For the wages of sin is death; but the gift of God is eternal life through Jesus Christ our Lord (KJV)*. Some people will go to any length to have sexual relations. Some people don't know this, but a private sexual moment on the internet is still sex. People have explored different methods of sex for personal satisfaction as if they were in the Sexology field of study. There are drugs of all sorts to make the encounter last longer or be more exciting. Why can't we see that Satan has taken this beautiful creation of God and polluted it? As Christians we need to understand that each time we have sexual intercourse with a different partner we carry a part of each one with us. If your sex partner encountered sex with a bi-sexual in the past, when the two of you have sex you are having sex with your partner's partners and the bi-sexual person's partners. Sex is not a game nor is it a contest to determine, "Who is the best" or "who have been with the most partners." It is not recreational.

This is the method God chose for reproduction. Reproduction cannot take place between two men or two women. It is also an ordained act between husband and wife. God created sex; therefore, it is good. He even instructs the husband and the wife not to abstain from sex for long periods of time or Satan will try to tempt one or the other. It is an intimate togetherness that makes them one and God is pleased. Conversely, if a couple is not married, but is sexually active, it is very unpleasant before the Lord. This is living in sin and out of fellowship with God. Is sex so good that you are willing to risk your health or life for it? Someone once said, "I live for sex." This is a dangerous person because it shows that he will engage in sex with whoever will give her body to him. Having pubic lice won't matter to this sex craved person. Sexual greed will cause a person to engage in sex with another individual carrying an STD (as long as there is a drug to cure it). Don't be so fast to lose your virginity or self-respect to this sex hungry world. Keep yourself clean of sexual sin.

Lust Causes Corruption:

Galatians 6:8 For he that soweth to his flesh shall of the flesh reap corruption; but he that soweth to the Spirit shall of the Spirit reap life everlasting.

There is a lesson to be learned in this world we live in. It mainly deals with prosperity, industries, and self-satisfaction. The industries of this world that are owned and managed by people who have the mentality of always moving forward at any cost. Owners of these mega businesses will go to great lengths to be the most profitable organization. Putting sexuality on the front line is the rule, not the exception. We must avoid being affected by these influences. Think of what effect posing half dressed on a billboard or in a magazine would have on you. We must respect ourselves to obtain respect from others. Furthermore, the pictures or images will be around long after you've married and started a family. Is it worth the embarrassment to escalate into adulthood and have the pictures creep back into your life and be viewed by your spouse or children? Sexual exploitation is a money making industry that can hurt the lives both male and female. Many young adults are willing to take risks to move up in the world fast, but fail to see the big picture. We all have to make our own choices in life, but we often fail to think before we act. It's understandable, but not acceptable how young minds can be caught up in taking high risks and accepting what appears to be the opportunity of a life time, only to later discover that it wasn't an opportunity but a trap. To live life in regret is not living a fulfilled life. Worldly people live by the standards of doing whatever it takes with no regards to morals, but Christians have an image to maintain. *Romans 8:5* tells us, *For they that are after the flesh do mind the things of the flesh; but they that are after the Spirit the things of the Spirit (KJV).* Once we were saved we became new creatures through Christ Jesus. Therefore, we must imitate Christ's life as much as possible. This means dressing moderately, marrying within biblical standards, speaking with clean words and not profanity or filthy language. It's understood that teenagers like to have fun but for too many sex has become a part of that fun. Their thought process is, "Why not make money while doing what's most enjoyable?" Even more so, "Why not get a promotion or my dream job while having fun?" One answer…you earned that promotion by being a prostitute. Solution, earn what you get; otherwise it's not an achievement. Again, it falls back to sin. The way that you get the job is the way you will have to keep it. This may call for being sexual with others to keep the job. After years have past, you may have established some stability, but no job security because the career was based on sexual favors. Everyone in the office knows; therefore, if you leave it is unlikely you will receive a favorable reference. You may have acquired years of experience, but unable to be recognized for it. Don't build a life on negative behaviors because it's bad business.

The key to sexual purity begins with the renewing of your mind and the determination to keep yourselves free from sexual sin. Celibacy is a strange word for the world, which explains why sex sells. Almost every aspect of television has turned to sex in some form or fashion to maintain its business. Commercials of all types are geared towards sex. Many actors and actresses can't find a moral movie to take part in because so many movies require sexual scenes or nudity. Actors are now disrespecting their wives because the money is in sexual roles to entertain their viewers. Young girls are taking off their clothes to obtain a leading role and men are indulging in their vulnerability.

There is a tremendous amount of lust in the world, and the industries are banking on it. The very thing that is making them rich is destroying us as a people. We can control this situation; however, we are allowing it to control us. Sexual roles in the television industry are almost mandatory. That's what sells; therefore, actors and actresses must play these roles if they want a job. Unfortunately, for many it is the career of choice. To be taken in by a society that feeds off sexual lust is absolutely a low point in a person's life. There has to be a turning point, and there is one that starts with you and me. Take a stand for Christ and be the example for someone who needs a mentor. Everyone is not a part of the sick things our society introduces. Fashions are too revealing and they are worn by teenage celebrities to capture the attention of young people. These industries focus on teenage interests then use them to build their empires. For this reason many teens are always looking for the latest fad. Businesses are aware of this and no matter how sexually suggestive a style may be, there will always be a market for it. Some people will support a new fashion with no regards to morals. Christians and religious people take these ideas into the house of God. Many of these choices have to do with maturity in life and their level of Christianity. Christianity is a growing process; therefore, we must learn about truth to obtain knowledge for daily living.

Clothes, conversation, our surroundings, and music can all affect the way we view sex. To daydream or imagine sexual encounters is sin. In addition, it makes it easier to fall when the opportunity presents itself. The body reacts to whatever is embedded within the mind just as the mind delivers whatever is in the heart. Our heart is the root of who we are no matter how we pretend to be something or someone else. We can be influenced by our surroundings; therefore we should seek change from God through Jesus Christ by the Holy Spirit. If you are a prostitute you don't have to be. If you have casual sex partners for whatever reason or even out of obligation it doesn't have to be that way. Change your thought process, your company, your music, television shows, or anything that promotes negative views or behaviors, especially those that consist of sexual intentions. Sexually active people will justify their behavior to relieve themselves of a guilty conscience, which is why anyone seeking a change must distance themselves from that influence. Sadly, we are sometimes torn by loved ones who support fornication and adultery. This doesn't make it right, but when there are carnal minded pastors and relatives encouraging such actions, it makes it harder to turn away, especially if it's already a struggle for you.

It's almost like everyone will be against you if you turn to godliness. What do you do? Pray. Ask God to give you strength to walk away with the courage to stand and remain faithful to that choice. Being successful and getting through it is based on your faith in God to deliver you and whether you are sincere about making a change. This may include ending the relationship with your female or male friend. It might not be easy if you've grown in love with this person, but remember if this person is meant for you, sex isn't the thing that's keeping you together. Cease from fornication and allow God to work in that area of your life. When you find the right person you will be loved for who you are within. Sex doesn't keep anyone from leaving unless it's the only reason they are there.

Breaking Free

John 8:36 If the Son therefore shall make you free, ye shall be free indeed (KJV).

Maintaining sexual purity can be a struggle for some of us. Some of us might not know this, but sex can become an addiction just as smoking, alcoholism, drugs, and others. To break any addiction first requires admittance of the problem. If the problem doesn't exist in the mind the individual can't see a need to be free from anything. Secondly, there must be a will of mind to take the necessary steps to break free. Any addiction is mental bondage that has convinced the body that it cannot survive unless it receives what has taken hold of it. Thirdly, seek outside help through counseling at church, a spiritual family friend, or mentor. If there is a close bond with the parent(s) they would be first choice. Lastly, (and they all work together as one) prioritize, focus, and follow through. Be consistent in counseling sessions to maintain a strong will to finish the course. In this process it might include eliminating certain friends, activities, movies, or anything that will naturally pull at you or hinder your progress. You may be strong, but hanging out with friends that are still active in sexual behaviors will eventually draw you in. Take this scenario for instance: You can't get dry if you don't come out of the rain. Once you're dry your thought process is better to make wise choices. Either use an umbrella (wisdom), or wear a raincoat (control), or don't go back out in the rain. Your common knowledge works as well, meaning, come from among your weaknesses until you are strong enough to resist them or just take them out of your life all together.

Sex can be controlling if it is a weakness. Once the urge arises it is the only thing on your mind. "Who to have sex with and how to make this happen," consume the thought process. Therefore, it has to be controlled or it will control you. Think about it, a rapist for example could have a wife to engage in sex as often as he likes, but his sexual addiction tells him that force is the only way he can get the most out of it. His sexual passions control his thought process and lead him into many sexual assaults to fulfill the lust that his mind tells his body he needs. So he thrives on it day and night watching and waiting for his next victim.

Teenage years are one of the most challenging stages in the lives of youth, because at that age the body is changing, and the hormone level increases. They are not sure of how to handle it except to fulfill the hunger for sex. *I Corinthians 6:13 Meats for the belly, and the belly for meats…Now the body is not for fornication, but for the Lord; and the Lord for the body (KJV).* In many cases it doesn't matter who fulfill the need, just as long as the passion is satisfied. This bisexual behavior is known as, Pansexual. This is bad for both male and female, because there are adults who know about these changes taking place and seek after them to please their own sexual desires. It's enough that you have to deal with growing up, but for older men and women to have the audacity to approach a child for sexual favors is a disgrace. Don't be taken in by their kind words to entice you into taking whatever they can from you, which is your sexual purity. "Fresh meat" is what they call you, not even acknowledging that you are a person. Some of these sex offenders are married, but out of greed, they have a desire to make you used goods. They will persuade you to give up your virginity and/or use you just for sexual pleasures. Just so you will know, this is against the law, but they will try to convince you that they love you. Don't fall for it or believe for a minute that they will leave their husband or wife for you. They are only after sex! Keep yourselves…for you are worth more than what they are trying to make you out to be.

How can we maintain control when the desires rush in from no where? How do we over come the sexual emotions and urges when there hasn't been any temptation? These times are challenging as well mostly because our guard is down. These could also be the most dangerous times, because it could occur when the opportunity is present. The best way would be getting out of the situation or creating some type of distraction. Find something else to do differently that would lead your focus towards something that is totally non-sexual. Remove any sexual thoughts quickly, because the longer we dwell on them the harder it will be to be rid of them. The quicker we change our thought process the easier it will be to walk away from the situation. Overcoming sudden urges is a mental recovery. Prayer works and for physical distraction exercise or anything that changes the present setting.

Controlling the forces of this passion will be next to impossible if we don't have a desire to abstain from participation. To know we need to practice abstinence and to want to practice it is not the same. To say, "I know abstinence is godly living, but I enjoy sex," is knowledge without will. Sex is a natural part of life, but within the boundaries of marriage. With everything in us we have to aim for this approach in life. Otherwise, we will satisfy every sexual desire that we are faced with. For unbelievers, sex is a fun thing to do to satisfy a need, but as a Christian it's much more. Sin takes us out of fellowship with God, which means there is no communion or access to Him. Only when we confess our sins will the Savior, Jesus Christ, restore our relationship with God.

I John 2:1 My children, these things write I unto you, that ye sin not. And if any man sin, we have an advocate with the Father, Jesus Christ the righteous (KJV). So you can see that there is more to lose than the unbeliever. They are not a part of the Body of Christ; therefore, when they die their soul is bound for hell.

Hell is the worst possible end result for anyone, but remember it was an individual choice to reject Christ to accept a lesser reward which are pleasures of this world. To understand this concept, an unbeliever can't really sin to the point that it will affect their eternal destination. Sin can only cause them physical harm due to STDs, but their spiritual life won't be affected. This is why those who fail to believe in Jesus Christ live a carnal minded lifestyle with no sense of concern. Their life is all about pleasure of the body and obtaining material things. Prosperity is the focus of many people even some Christians are caught up in carnal thinking, but unbelievers concern is only about what happens here on earth. Life after death is not a concern of theirs. Children of God have to remain faithful to the choice we have made and not allow the lifestyle of others to change who we are. Unbelievers fail to realize the prince of this earth (Satan) works day and night to keep them in their mind-set and try to turn us from truth.

As humans we all have a need or want for something. Our desires might not be the same, but the want of spirituality, material assets, or physical fulfillment is still there in all of us. Many people spend their entire lives trying to make the connection to meet those needs. Anticipation lingers in the minds of those waiting for that special place and time to receive what is expected. During the wait to get a husband or wife, we can often lose patience. Lust creeps in from out of nowhere to convince us that we don't have to wait. To our advantage, lust can only be harmful if it is a part of our lives. In that we have a choice to obey it or reject it. When the body lusts after sex we don't have to obey it if we have the power of God in us. We can be in charge of our own lives and not allow sin to rule over us. Once sexual lust takes over it will convince the mind to justify its action. Lust has a purpose, which is to be satisfied. It doesn't want an explanation of why it exists, how to prevent it, nor where it came from. Lust is a desire that wants to be fed; therefore, we must not take it in as a part of our lives. Learning to resist it is the key to remain in control of it. *I Peter 2:11 … abstain from freshly lusts, which war against the soul; (KJV).*

We must also be mindful of the relationships that we are involved in. Consider a Christian seeking a relationship with an unbeliever. There will be a clash in characters, and they will voice many different opinions. How can two walk together except they agree? The conflict is night (unbeliever) and day (Christian), which has no fellowship one with the other. How can day and night dwell in the same place at the same time? This example does not say that dawn or sunset puts them at a compromise. Day implies the peak hours and night implies the darkest hours. Although each serves its purpose, these two are not in unison. The moon and the sun are not working together in the same place at one given time. Christians and unbelievers cannot spiritually walk together, it's like oil and water; they don't mix. *I Corinthians 6:14 Be ye not unequally yoked together with unbelievers: for what fellowship hath righteousness with unrighteousness? and what communion hath light with darkness?(KJV)*

Another failure waiting to happen is dating a married person. We must first be realistic to realize that a married person has no intentions on divorcing his or her spouse for you, especially a teenager. And if he or she does, who's to say this person won't do the same to you when the next good thing walks by? Chances are this person is looking for additional sexual pleasures, which undoubtedly could be found at home. Greed is a good word to describe these selfish-minded individuals. Don't lower your standards to meet the desires of adulterers. You sometimes feel unloved or unwanted by your peers, so you turn to the arms of anyone that you feel will fulfill what you long for or to complete the empty space inside. For a while you feel that it is working, but when your heart falls for this person he or she will end the relationship, which puts the emptiness back, along with a broken heart. If you examine this situation, you will discover that the emptiness never truly left. To meet with a person once a week for sexual encounters, a few words to entice the mind, and some caress to keep the body wanting more is nothing more than being charmed. Once the evening is over, you'll return to your empty bed, and this person will go to bed with her husband or with his wife. Have you really been relieved of loneliness? No. Temporary sexual satisfaction is not fulfillment. It's just physical pleasure with no meaning, no completeness, nor inner fulfillment. If inner fulfillment is what you are seeking, don't allow anyone to waste your time with lies. At your age, you should be seeking personal goals you might have and enjoying life. Not seeking after love relationships that might not last due to career choices and the many opportunities that lies await for you. Focus towards building on your strengths and work toward achieving them. In all things keep your mind on God to lead you through the difficult circumstances and decisions you might face in life.

Furthermore, consider your spirituality in the eyes of others. Not adding pressure, but it is our duty to present ourselves as living witnesses of who Jesus is. We are spiritual beings existing on this earth by way of the physical body. Our spirit is of God; therefore, we must keep the body clean of any sin. Our spirit is who we are and not the body. We spend a lot of time making sure that our outer appearance is groomed and pleasant for the eyes of others, but our major concern should be with the inner man. Are we feeding our spirit with biblical knowledge to obtain strength to resist sin? Physical appearance is good: therefore, we should exercise, eat healthy, maintain personal hygiene, and dress conservatively. We must also eat the word of God for spiritual growth and to maintain a loving spirit toward one another and dress our mind every day in godliness to conduct ourselves properly. The spiritual and physical beings need to be presented in a way that God is pleased. Also, let us love people for who they are and not based on their outward appearance. Deception has destroyed many people in the name of artificial love. The outward appearance will change, which is why we should love the inner man.

When selecting a mate for marriage at that point of your life, always investigate the soul of that person. The outer reflection may be irresistible, but the inner self may be an advocate of the devil. Once marriage takes place that individual is yours. Whatever or whoever he or she may be. Pray before making decisions in life. God will lead you in the right direction and detour you from the wrong ones.

We should make choices that are good for both the mind and body to avoid stressing ourselves and tearing ourselves down. Our being consists of spirit and body, which war against each other daily. We must remain focused to view the big picture of life. To live a here and now lifestyle will always end up in regret. Sex might be enjoyable to the body, but outside of marriage it wars against the soul. As Christians, we can't allow this temporary emotion to determine our eternal destination. The feeling comes, it's satisfied, and there's the feeling of living in the regret. Is it truly worth the disrespect, shame, and immorality that come with the act? The end result could be a conceived child, a sexually transmitted disease, or worse an incurable transmitted disease.

Teenage pregnancy is hard to face or deal with. Although, it might be an inconvenience we can't take a life out of convenience. As Christians we must take responsibility for our actions. There is no running from them, covering them, nor ignoring them. Everyday of our lives we are faced with the choice between good and evil. The choice we make is the choice we have to live with. Abortion is only an option when it endangers the life of the mother. Of course, the world's point of view concerning this issue is different. In spite of secular views, life does begin at conception.

There are many issues that we face as individuals as well as a country due to the abuse and misuse of sex. To some people it is a hobby, to others it's a stress rellever. It's just a fun thing to do for a lot of people and it's an addiction to many others. This beautiful thing God created for husband (man) and wife (woman) has become a tool for businesses. What happened to respecting ones self? Our bodies are not toys for any man who wants to play, nor is a man's body an object for women to indulge. We must respect ourselves, because if we don't no one else will.

Young ladies, guys will play if we allow them. Young men, females will use you if you allow them. There are males and females who want to be mature young men and women, but not sure of how to accomplish such a goal. The simple fact is some people were never taught; therefore, they live by the only lifestyle they've ever known. Remember that you don't have to become a part of someone else's tangled web. Fortunately, some people are blessed with godly influences to give them a different view of life. This is why it is so important that Christians are in fellowship with God at all times. We never know when God will put someone in our lives to be a positive influence. Just because someone comes from a bad background doesn't mean that destruction will be his or her end. We have to take charge of our lives by putting God first which means living by His word and studying the bible for biblical wisdom and knowledge. The more we know about who God is the closer to him we will become.

Smooth talkers and charmers shouldn't persuade us to do things that we know are wrong. Being sexually active to keep a boyfriend or girlfriend is self-deception. If sex is the only thing keeping the relationship, then it isn't a relationship built off love. These types of relationships struggle to last. It's totally physical and if that's the only thing holding the relationship together anyone can step in and tear it down. Don't be taken in by individuals who make you feel obligated to have sex. Relationships should be based on trust, loyalty, honesty, and a great deal of patience and sacrifice. Don't settle for anything just to say that you have someone. Keep your bodies pure and free of sexual sin and glorify God in your body which is the temple of God once being saved.

Teen Pregnancy And Marriage

Marriage is serious and should not be taken lightly. When we fall in love for the first time, we feel like, "This is the one." We devote everything to the relationship and many times marriage is not far away. There are many things to consider before marriage; furthermore, there are many things we haven't learned about ourselves at the young age of eighteen. Marriage comes with sacrifice, patience, and trust. At such a young age there hasn't been time to explore life on your own. Your entire life was under the leadership of your parents or guardians; therefore, you need time for self-development. Even if it means a few years of college before actually taking vows that are meant to last the rest of your lives. To marry directly out of high school might cause frustration and irritation. Some people have survived it, but many have not. Accepting each others differences is a challenge within itself. In high school during the dating game differences are cute and funny. When you are married and have live with those differences everyday, they won't be quite as cute and certainly not funny. A few stable-minded individuals have made it, but rushing into marriage without biblical counseling can end up in divorce. Not only personal issues, but managing money can be a major conflict if both persons involved are not in agreement. Remember the following:

- Always put God first

- Know what it would take to stay together

- Take the time to learn each other

- Counseling is a great idea from a pastor and money manager or financial advisor.

Should a couple marry if there is a baby involved? No! Never marry out of obligation or just because a baby was conceived, especially if there isn't stability in the relationship. Just wait until God leads you in that direction.

Pregnancy can be a challenge at an early age. Being a parent has to come into play for the child's sake even if you are not ready. There are many mentors such as pastors, teachers, or great leaders but these are not replacements of parents being mentors in their child's life. A child's development will mature more effectively by seeing responsibility, devotion, spiritual structure, and leadership on a daily basis.

As parents, we often teach our children not to do wrong and tell them where bad decisions will lead. So, they develop the concept that parents are perfect. As we teach them on their level, it's good to let them know that we have made some mistakes growing up. The most important factor is teaching them truth, which is biblical knowledge and being the example in their lives. They sometimes stray as they grow, but continue living and teaching in God's will. The bible teaches us that love never fails; therefore, always let them know that they are loved, but never support their bad choices. Our job is to teach them truth, but the ultimate choice will be theirs. If they choose to make bad choices, don't stop loving them, just continue in truth and allow them to face the consequences of their choices. Just as your parent(s) have done and are doing with you.

Sometimes teenagers seek fulfillment in a child. They allow loneliness to lead them into a sexual relationship with plans to become pregnant. The decision to have a baby at an immature age is not a wise choice. A child should be raised by both a mother and a father. Furthermore, planning to become a single teen parent is a selfish act. Without an education how can a teen properly support a child? Also consider the child's needs which should always come first. Looking to a child to feel complete or to fill the emptiness will blind this person to the child's emotional needs. Family was God's plan; therefore, planning a family should be done God's way.

Making Choices

Jealousy appears to move teenagers in a negative direction, in some cases they have turned to violence. Reacting to jealousy that causes harm to another individual is not an act of love, its rage. *Psalms 6:34 For jealousy is the rage of a man: therefore he will not spare in the day of vengeance (KJV).* In many cases it's an impulsive act that leads to a traumatic end. The attack is on one person, but the results will affect many. This is a selfish reaction, which is solely based on rejection and a way to seek revenge. *Romans 12:19 Dearly beloved, avenge not yourselves, but rather give place unto wrath: for it is written, Vengeance is mine; I will repay, saith the Lord (KJV).* Before acting on non-sense, think about the rest of your life. This is one boy or girl that will not bring an end to your world if you are not with him or her. There will be someone else, so don't throw away your entire life for anyone. The pain that you may be feeling at that time may seem unbearable, but think of the consequences before doing something that can't be undone. Think of the people that will be affected, most importantly, remember that you are a Christian; therefore, base your decision on, "What would Jesus do?" Just walk away from the situation and resist evil thoughts. *1 Thessalonians 5:15 See that none render evil for evil unto any man; but ever follow that which is good, both among yourselves, and to all men (KJV).* Jealousy over someone sleeping around isn't worth losing your education, self-respect, or your freedom.

There are sayings, "Love makes you do things that you never thought you would do," and "All for the sake of love," some might say. "I love you too much to see you with someone else," dwell in the inner most thoughts of many. You might think this is cute, but being with someone who thinks like this could make a turn for the worse.

Those of us who believe in the Lord Jesus Christ as being the Son of God know there is life after death. Therefore, live the life of a Christian in order to receive eternal life. Christians cannot allow unbelievers to change our view of life to practice sin willfully. God is faithful and just to forgive our sins, but to practice sin with the mind-set of unconditional forgiveness is not the mind of a spiritual Christian. *Romans 6:1-2 What shall we say then? Shall we continue in sin, that grace may abound? God forbid…(KJV).* To live in the form of Christianity or to be religious as a tradition will allow false godliness to please the eyes and not the will of God. Christianity is not about pleasing people, but to be pleasing to God. In order to know what is expected of us by God, we must study our bible daily or as often as possible. The bible is a map to direct us in the path of life. It's also a mirror to show us where we have made bad choices and how to turn away from them. In our spiritual life, the bible will teach us to take one day at a time. The bible also encourages, give strength, as well as the wisdom needed to survive among the evils of this world. The more we study, the closer we will be drawn to God, which provide courage to stand on truth. The will to do the right thing has to be an individual choice. Not to impress or to please others, but it's who we have chosen to be. Failure to believe that God is who he said he is does not change his identity. He is God whether people believe it or not. Therefore, we must learn the truth for ourselves and not take the word of others. To believe just by hearing will make it easy for an unbeliever to influence and change your thinking, because it's not rooted. If we study for ourselves to learn of Jesus Christ who died for our sins, we will build a relationship with him to view life through his eyes, and it will give us the foundation that cannot be destroyed by anyone. Once we have this concept, pleasing the world won't be a priority in our lives, nor will pleasing the flesh through sin, because of our renewed minds. When we change our mind-set from carnal to spiritual, life will become so much clearer, and it will make us stronger. We can't allow ourselves to be caught-up in worldly pleasures because it takes us out of fellowship with God. Let's encourage our friends to do the right thing and not allow them to pull us into doing the wrong thing(s).

There is so much more to life than sex. Many teenagers want to have fun, which consist of sex, parties, sex, hanging out, sex, drinking, sex, drugs, sex, sports, and more sex. Sex appears to be the source of making all fun things enjoyable. Sex seems to put the "F" in fun. Being sexy also plays a major role in teen life. Conversely, males don't groom as much as females, but females flock to them in spite of their appearance or image. It's all physical and not mentally reasonable. For instance, girls wear their clothes too tight and boys wear their clothes too big. This is not logical. Therefore, teenagers are encouraged to expand their thought process. In many cases rational thinking is limited, is this you? Only seeing what is wanted and not having a desire to think beyond that. The "fun" life has not consumed just the sexual aspects of life, but it has now affected education.

Life is so much fun until education is being substituted with a GED. There isn't a shortcut to a fulfilled life, but it has become the norm to some teenagers. The family-oriented minds are fading. Values have been disregarded.

The very things that made a man a man and a woman a woman are being redefined by society and the government. Whatever makes life convenient is the new way; therefore, hard work and values are losing ground. Young people, you are not inferior, but if you continue on this path many of you will be labeled then classified as second best. Open your eyes and see what's happening around you. Those of you that won't lose your life to STDs will be taken by the system or killed. All in the name of fun many of you will miss the real joy of life. Fun is good in its place and when it's in line with cleanliness, honesty, godliness, and others that don't require sin.

So many individuals have a belief of "A way out," which motivates or influence their thinking and persuade them into participating in sexual activities. Pharmaceuticals and researchers have provided the understanding that STDs can be cured, treated, or maintained for a period of time. Sexually driven minds rejoice on this type of information. As long as there is a hint of a chance to recover from an STD the will to practice is present.

For some people, fun isn't fun unless the body is intoxicated or drugged illegally. They have convinced themselves that sex isn't good unless it's under those conditions. What they fail to realize is that those conditions make sexual activities more dangerous. Drugs and alcohol remove logical thinking which make you subject to any opportunity presented to you. The willingness to engage in sex becomes an act of foolish behaviors. Many times more than two partners are interacting together. Orgies contribute to STDs spreading more rapidly. Sadly, those newly affected don't know who gave them the disease. If these fun parties are done regularly, there is no assurance of anything because anything can happen.

Seniors leave home and start college during the fall to discover a number of sexual evils lurking around campus. Be wise and never forget what you were taught on self respect at home. Hold on to spiritual wisdom and keep your body pure. Don't be deceived by smooth talkers and beware of charmers. Before you hear what he or she has to say, examine his or her life to see whether it's good or bad.

Image

Everyone has his or her own personality (as well as we all should); however, we are often impressed by the characteristics of someone else. Whether it's how he or she handles life situations or his or her drive to be successful. Maybe it's their moral status or temperance. Whatever it is, we take a likeness to it and dream of being like them someday. Sometimes we fail to realize that someone is looking at us in the exact or similar ways. Therefore, we must conduct ourselves in a way that won't lead them into immorality. We often believe that our sexual life is our own private business, and it is, but it should be within the boundaries of marriage. Otherwise, it shouldn't be a part of us. If we do, we come across as hypocrites, and our lifestyle have no effect on Christian living. This is displeasing to God, because we are here to live in the image of Jesus Christ. He lived the example for us to follow and we are to mimic His life on earth.

The double mindedness of individuals allow them to believe that hypocrisy is okay as long as it's hidden from public knowledge. Others have the mind-set of spiritual elimination justifies sexual sin. These assumptions are wrong. We will either be Christians or pretenders. Christians have a different aspect on spiritual life than unbelievers. We have an obligation to live according to the Word of God. Sexual sin to us is not only against God, but against our own bodies. Sin that's committed in the flesh must be repaid in the flesh. Sometimes our physical illnesses are not trials. Sometimes we have to look back at the lives we've lived to determine if we are simply reaping what we've sown. We bring many things on ourselves then ask, "Why did God allow this to happen to me?" Abstinence does not guarantee that we won't face sickness, but sexual sin won't be the cause of certain illnesses or misfortunes. There will be trials and tests that are not related to sickness or physical disabilities. We must be faithful to our choice to be a Christian and trust in God to see us through the journey of this temporary life.

Turn away from those things that pull at our sexual passions, whether it's music, certain clothes, individuals, or movies. Whatever it is that hinders us from sexual purity, should be avoided. At first it might be difficult, but prioritizing and staying focused will make it easier.

We shouldn't be caught up in the world's logic of what is acceptable and what is not acceptable. The prostitute or exotic dancer might say, "I need money, and I have what it takes to make the exchange." This is not logical, but it is a secular point of view that is degrading and eliminates self worth. Don't allow the world to define who you are. Once you are no longer valuable to them, they will disregard you. Know who you are as a Christian and live by those standards. Sitcoms, movies, and music make fornication appear legitimate, but wrong cannot be justified. Young minds are often taken advantage of by deception. Manipulating your thoughts to believe that heterosexuality is a thing of the past, transforming your bodies into what's considered sexy to reveal to the world, and living together unmarried is better than being tied down. Take the initiative to learn truth then apply it. We are who we choose to be and not what others say we are. You are not to be used or made into used goods. For instance, a dinner date isn't repaid by a night of sexual favors. This is still prostitution. Any exchange of sex for money, dinner, or anything of small or great value is prostitution. Yes, this includes a prom date.

If we say that we are Christians, but live our lives with lustful eyes, how can we be in unity with God? If our clothes are too revealing and our lifestyle is in-sink with the world, how can we be in-sink with God? Being in agreement with God means living by his standards, which might not be in agreement with friends, but our loyalty is to Jesus Christ. With this in mind, what do we choose to keep, a secular reputation or Christian morals? The answer lies within the resulting end of the choice. Secularism will result in everlasting damnation and Christianity leads to eternal life with God.

Some people believe that if they commit to Christ, they can no longer have fun and from that time forward life would be boring. This is not true. Fun depends on how it is defined by that individual. Fun for some is drinking, clubbing, smoking, cursing, etc. Others might define fun as sporting activities, games, family gatherings, etc. Some might even define fun as any event that makes them laugh. Joy in the Lord is fun for many. Fun is a combination of things, but godliness pertains to those things that don't defile the body, nor corrupt ones thinking, or condemn the soul. Therefore, being saved doesn't take away recreational fun, because God put them here for our enjoyment.

Homosexuality/lesbianism

The controversy of homosexuality and lesbianism falls between Christian believers and non-believers. Same sex relationships are more than an act against marital guidelines; it's an act against nature. This country was founded on the grounds of Christianity and to allow unbelievers to bring conflict against the country's foundation is a sign of weakness in leadership. Not to mention the dangers it place on the country. Anyone who builds on faith in God only to reject Him once it has been established can expect persecution. The bible speaks against homosexuality and lesbianism in the Old and New Testament. Two cities were destroyed by God due to this unnatural act.

These sins are becoming the norm in our society; although it's not a law in most states to recognize same sex marriage, they are taking a large portion of everyday norms such as: television, local church assemblies, businesses, etc. and planting themselves in the mist of them. Older adults might not accept it, but the target is the younger generation. Making homosexuality and lesbianism the choice of their future by making it a norm for them by the time they reach adulthood. This is their approach to pass same sex marriage laws throughout the United States. Scientists are already researching animals with the assumption that some species of the same sex can reproduce which makes it possible for humans of the same sex to reproduce. Insisting on studies to create the possibility of same sex reproduction is absolutely ridiculous. Young people, the world is making a turn for the worse and the initiators are depending on you to make it happen. Don't work against the plan of God to accomplish the very thing that will eventually destroy you. Don't be blinded by the evil things that ungodly individuals are trying to bring to pass. Keep your mental and physical being free of destruction that man is bringing on themselves unknowingly. The choices we make in life are the choices we have to live with. Therefore, we can't allow others to create definitions to make good bad and bad good. Example: Marriage is good, but it's made to be bad; therefore, many have chosen to live together unmarried. Homosexuality was frowned upon and those who did it hid it. Now they are trying to obtain the same rights as godly marriages. Man and woman don't want to be married, but the homosexuals do, where is the logic in that? Please stay focused on truth and don't allow foolish ideas and/or laws to be justified in your minds.

We have to take responsibility of our own lives. Regardless of the situation, there has to be guidelines in our behavior. Neither counseling, nor moving to another location, nor lectures will put our lives in perspective if we haven't made the choice to change within. There are many difficult decisions to make; then there is the process of following through. Therefore, self discipline plays a major role in actual change. The biggest problem of making change is to stop relying on self and depend on God. Satan is a powerful force, and we cannot face this force without the almighty God. When we try to stand on our own might, we will fall every time, because alone, we are no match to Satan. Through Christ we can do all things, but without Him we can do nothing. *John 15:5 I am the vine, ye are the branches: He that abideth in me, and I in him, the same bringeth forth much fruit: for without me ye can do nothing (KJV).* Change is hard for adults, but it is a tremendous challenge for young adults. Denying self to proceed in the direction of Jesus Christ takes a lot of courage. Teenagers today feel the need to impress their friends or to always finish on top. Unfortunately, the ones trying to build the impressive image are the ones that end up in trouble. We might be influenced by peers, but the ultimate choice is ours. We can't blame others for our short comings because we have to search ourselves for the source of our problems. Whether we admit it or not, the roots of our problems are inside of us. Denial can and will prevent us from overcoming these issues in our lives. We can sometime become our own worst enemy. To continue in unfortunate events and to never resolve the issue from within will keep us blaming others for our decision to be sexually active outside of marriage.

Accepting responsibility of our actions is only half the battle. Seeking the proper help to improve our lifestyle is just as important. Many times, people view life as if it was created just for them. No one is promised tomorrow, but the lifestyles of so many people say that they have forever. They don't take life seriously, just living it through and going through the motions. It appears that the purpose of our being doesn't seem to matter much in today's society.

You need to know that you are not a product of society nor are you a product of your environment. Take charge of your life and become who God says you are. Be mindful that society have a number of industries to up hold, and they will target whomever with whatever it takes to sell the product. Don't be caught up in this madness that only cares about the dollar. You are better than that and don't allow anyone else to tell you otherwise. For instance, the norm for secularism is, "It's just music." Whether we can see it or not, whatever we listen to, or whatever information you are exposed to on a regular basis, will become a part of you. Once the mind is exposed to certain things, it becomes acceptable and soon it is a lifestyle for some, but tolerated by others. After a period of time you will date people of this character or become a fornicator yourself. Whatever you consume, will eventually come out. Therefore, feed your spirit with godliness and godliness will become you.

We don't have to go about trying to make others see Christ in us, because if we just live by biblical standards, it will be known. Our perspective should be founded on our origin, which is, we are created beings of God. Our original purpose was to dwell on the earth forever, but sin broke the connection with God and man. Jesus came to earth to reconcile man back to God through his death on the cross and his resurrection on the third day. Now our purpose is to help unbelievers accept Jesus Christ as his or her personal savior, by confessing hope in Christ. Christians have a responsibility to live in obedience to be the example for others to see Christ in us. Christianity is no longer the way of the world, but it has now been transformed to the term, "Lifestyle." Society has mentally placed God in a box to only access when there is trouble. They have redefined

God to be someone who will never allow tragedies or death. Society seeks to deceive weak minded people to believe that everyone is saved and that Jesus isn't the only way to get to heaven. They also do this by promoting homosexuality, lesbianism, and have legalized living together unmarried. This sin has been given a new name to justify its existence, which is called "Common Law Marriage." A more common and truthful name for it is, "Shacking-up."

It's hard, but not impossible to live under today's stress and pressures of life. But... everyone that you associate with is having worldly fun and nothing has happened to them. So, you wonder if you are missing out in vain. These thoughts can lead you into taking dangerous risks and chances that you normally wouldn't take. It's easy to be distracted with assumptions from a lack of knowledge. The imagination can go wild with just a little misunderstanding. This isn't only true with young people, but adults as well. We must be careful in our thought process because it has led people to do the unthinkable. In regards to conflict, it can be avoided by communication. It would be a waste to spend precious time dwelling on thoughts that are not true or misunderstood. Once we begin to think negatively, it gets bigger and bigger. Before long, we will begin to act on our thoughts that may only exist in our minds. Communication is the key to eliminate responding in a hateful, harmful, or disrespecting way. Talking can answer questions before they become issues. The purpose of resolution is to keep peace. All of us have faced this dilemma at one point and time in our lives. The solution is learning how to deal with them.

Unresolved issues need to be handled immediately. The problems may consist of physical or mental abuse. Don't confuse assumptions with actuality in this matter. Sexual abuse should be dealt with from the start. Don't allow it to go on regardless of who your molester is. It might be embarrassing or not knowing the outcome if you report this person or it just may be frightening, but don't give anyone that kind of control or power over you. Keeping problems and/or unresolved issues inside will work against you and eventually affect your behavior. This is what shouldn't happen because the result could end up worst than you intended. Therefore, we should open up to someone regardless of what the situation is, whether it is sexual, mental, or physical abuse. There are cases such as mental depression or feeling as though everyone is against you. Don't keep these harmful feelings trapped inside. Pray and seek help from parent(s), a pastor, a local church family member, a trusting family member, or adult family friend of the same sex. There are also hotlines in different areas to take you out of abusive situation. God loves you, and you were not created to be violated by anyone. Male and female, don't ever believe that you deserve this type of cruelty. Pray and search deep within yourself for the will to break free then trust in God to deliver you. You are worth it and you can do it.

Self-Respect

Self-respect and abstinence are still in existence although society wants you to believe otherwise. Celibacy is a choice just as immorality. Regardless of the impact these types of messages have on us, the ultimate decision to live by them is ours. We will individually stand before God at the judgment, it's at that time when all of the choices we've made will matter. So, living to please man will make room for a special spot in the lake of fire. It's quite knowledgeable that the lake of fire seems unrealistic to many, maybe even something that might be seen on the Sci-Fi Channel. Such a place can't possibly exist or can even be imagined, but rest assured that it is real whether it is accepted or not. God's Word said it and if we believe in Him we believe his Word. God is real and just because some fail to believe that He is real doesn't change the fact that He is. *Hosea 4:6* teaches that, *My people are destroyed for lack of knowledge: (KJV)*. Many people often disrespect themselves by having multiple sex partners. Society today is willfully rejecting the knowledge of God and who He is. As Christians we know that there are promises of God.

The promises are not all good. If we fail to accept Jesus Christ as Lord or fail to live according to His Word, we will not inherit the Kingdom of Heaven. This is not only true with sexual sin, but any form of ungodly living. We must repent of our sins and turn away from them daily. A scenario of life on earth is like a recipe. We put in the ingredients of our lifestyle and once it's been baked by God, whatever comes out of the oven will determine your eternal resting place. So, as we look at our lives we should think carefully about what's going into the mixing bowl. One of the good things about God is that he gave us Jesus, which is an opportunity to receive a clean bowl when we give our life to Him. Therefore, when we fall short of His Word we can sincerely repent and we can still obtain a new start with Him. (Another scenario; in baking a cake that reflects young people wanting to grown up too fast. You can have all of the right ingredients in the cake, but baking it too fast will cause it to be firm on the outside, but too doughy on the inside. Your outer appearance shows that you are a young man or woman, but the inside may be still immature which makes you vulnerable for the evil one to detour you in the wrong direction. Be patient and continue to live by the rules of your parent(s), and in due time the inside will be as firm as the outside and you'll be ready to face the world on your own with the Lord on your side).

Old fables such as: "Enjoy your youth while you are young" or "you're only young once" are foolish sayings when it comes to sexual purity. Sure it's okay to enjoy youth activities, but to indulge in youthful lusts is a sinful act that could bring STDs or death.

There are young people who date married individuals. This is absolutely out of the question! Learn this fact of life while you are young so that it will not carry over into adulthood. Adults should not date children, teens, or young adults. Do not entertain sexual nor dating conversations with them. If there is one that is persistent, consult with a respectful adult to have this person reported. It is a known fact that some males seek young boys to engage in homosexuality and this is also true with young girls. Therefore, it is important to refrain from close intimate relationships with adults.

Some people have and some people still are disrespecting themselves by living with a person unmarried. Many individuals might debate this issue stating that it's not a sin; therefore, living under these conditions out of ignorance. A lack of respect is also associated with phone sex. Sexual immorality is not wrong in the eyes of the world, it's just a lifestyle. Sin is sin, but we must understand that living in sin isn't the same as committing sin. To willfully continue in a sinful act is living in sin, which cuts off the communication line with God. Sure we allow circumstances to put us in situations, but that doesn't justify our staying in sin. God is expecting us to conduct ourselves in the way that is pleasing to Him. If we say we are Christians, then we should live as Christians. If you say you are an unbeliever, then that lifestyle is expected of you. Make a choice and live by that choice. Once we chose to give our life to Jesus as Lord and Savior, we must remain faithful to that choice. This is the struggle with the undecided. Having a desire to be godly, but don't want to change lifestyles. Although the emphasis is on sexual sin, we should work toward omitting all sins to the best of our ability.

Sometimes our loved ones die in sin, and we so badly want them to be in heaven, but based on their lifestyle and spiritual fruit, they were out of fellowship with God. Once they are gone, we can't pray them to heaven nor hope them there. As individuals, we have to work while we are breathing, because once we die, it's over. Our eternal destination is already determined and there is no changing it.

Sexual purity carries a lot of weight. Although in our youth we view life differently. Others treat us based on the way we carry ourselves and bear witness to our character on how we respect ourselves. For instance, if a person approached you with a sexual slur as a form of compliment, you shouldn't respond. Don't recognize it with your eyes, a head turn, or gestures because once you do you've characterized yourself to be at that level with very little value.

Jesus, to unbelievers, is unrealistic and they refuse to view sexual purity as a moral issue even less so a sin. The concept of life on earth, in their opinion, is non-spiritual for most of them. Some say there is a God and after death we all go to heaven. Some believe there is no God and after death that's the end. Some don't have an opinion, they just know that they are here and that is what's important. This is why Christians can't allow unbelievers to make choices for us nor help us with a decision concerning our personal lives.

Correction will grieve those who hate to make a change for godliness. Truth is good for those who wish to follow it, but it will bring heartache to those who despise it. We know that fornication is wrong; therefore, we try to avoid situations that will pull at us. To despise this knowledge of truth makes it harder to obey. The mind begins to find ways to justify the sin, even though sin cannot be justified. We may have a reason for the choices we make, but it still doesn't change the fact that wrong can't be made right. The battle in our minds between right and wrong will tear us apart if we choose to reject truth. When we've done what we know is wrong, truth will still be there waiting to convict us of our sinful actions. It's easier to accept truth (the Word of God), instead of fighting against it which makes life harder. Temptation will be there, but we must prioritize our lives and stay focused. Friends who are not ready to live godly may sometime try to influence our choices. Having a mind of our own and not following after others, especially those misleading, will also make life easier.

Incest

Incest is a tremendous issue that requires immediate attention. What is incest? It is a sexual act between family members such as: Brother and sister, father and daughter, mother and son, father and son, or mother and daughter. Not excluding cousins, aunts, uncles, nieces, nephews, step-fathers, and step-mothers.

[During my research, I've read the confessions of brothers and sisters admitting the pleasures of experiencing sexual intercourse with their siblings. They expressed the excitement as well as their desire to do it again. Many of them were young adults which mean they were old enough to know better] Sister and brother should not engage in a sexual encounter nor enjoy it as if they were a couple. Neither should a parent and child seek sexual favors from one another. Many people have redefined sex in their minds to make it what they want it be. For some it is merely a method to satisfy sexual urges.

Statistics show high numbers of incest cases in the United States alone. Children by the millions around the world are victims of this heartless crime. They are afraid to tell anyone because their perpetrators have place fear in them; therefore, some children live in denial to escape reality. Others are traumatized to the degree of amnesia. Some may even bury the experience within themselves, which matures into a deep, revengeful anger that slowly eats away at them.

Don't be afraid to trust your parent(s) (if not the accused), a pastor, counselor, or teacher to report such activity. Just don't allow it to go on.

Regardless of the person who has molested you it is not your fault. This does not take away from your character or self-respect, but it diminishes theirs. Be encouraged, even during these bad times. Hold your head up and take the control away from this person. Go to the authorities to report the individual that is seeking sexual favors from you.

The worse case scenario is being molested by one parent with the other parent's acknowledgement but failing to do anything about it. Although this is a bad situation, it still doesn't mean you have to surrender. Don't allow these circumstances to place you in a mental prison or cause you to distance yourself for other people nor allow intimidation to become a part of you. Pray and ask God to lead you. *I Peter 5:7 Casting all your care upon him; for he careth for you. (KJV)*

Although incest in a sexual act outside of marriage the victim is not to blame. God will not hold you accountable for this crime because you haven't done anything wrong. So, if you are wondering how to restore your self-respect, you can't because you have never lost it. It was always there waiting for you to connect with it. Self-respect is inside of you and no one can take it from you...you'll have to give it away.

If you are a current victim of sexual abuse **R.A.I.N.N** *(Rape, Abuse, Incest National Network) is a non-profit organization that provides free confidential help seven days per week/twenty-four hours a day. Their hotline number is 800/656-HOPE. To read more about the organization log-on to* www.info@rainn.org

Incest is wrong and it doesn't matter if you are the perpetrator or a willing participant. I want to encourage you to take a look at yourself to determine your self-worth. You also, need to understand that sexual intimacy was designed for husband and wife. If you are the innocent party, seek help to be free of this person. If you are a willing participant or the perpetrator, you need to seek help to be delivered from your spiritual sickness.

Safe Sex

Is there such a thing as safe sex? That's the same as saying, "Steal, but don't get caught," or "Lie, but don't give it away." This is misleading information that will eventually catch-up with you. Safe sex? No.

There are some STDs that can be transmitted without ejaculation taking place. Using condoms during sex, removing the penis before ejaculation or any other method can guarantee protection from STD exposure. Abstinence is one of the only sure ways to avoid STDs. There are other ways to come in contact with STDs besides sexual intercourse. One way to be exposed to STDs is by kissing. It might seem harmless, but kissing a person who has been exposed to a STD through oral sex, can contract sexually transmitted diseases that hold the same affect. Diseases can also be transmitted by sharing a needle while doing drugs. This action is two disasters in one, so refrain from doing drugs as well.

Safe sex, what does that really mean? Fornication is okay as long as we are careful? Does it pertain to those who are going to do it any way? The truth about sex is the guidelines placed on the act. Wait until marriage, because any form of sexual activity before marriage is wrong.

If you have already participated in sexual activities, get tested to find out if you are infected. In the meantime, read available pamphlets to learn about STDs and how they could affect your body. Abstain from fornication from this point forward. Talk with friends to encourage them to abstain from fornication as well. Know the consequences of such sin and pray for strength to follow after righteousness. Identify yourself with the Lord and not the world. Increase your spiritual knowledge with the Word of God just as you increase your physical strength with food. Your body will die if you do not eat, so will your spirit grow cold to godliness without direction. The Word of God is your mirror to read and remove ungodliness from your life.

With every generation come different challenges of life. There are many statistics that identify STDs in its population based on gender, race, class, age, and so on, but due to statistical manipulation, let's not focus on these numbers just to put temporary fear in the mind to flock to a different group to practice the same sin. Instead, focus on the number infected regardless of race or gender. The fact is there are millions and millions of individuals infected with some type of STD. Many of them are not detected by sight; therefore, to be taken by a person's appearance doesn't guarantee a STD free individual. Sure he might be handsome, dresses nice, has a promising career, and live independently, but what does that really tell you? It only identifies with the external to say that he is doing well for himself. For example, let's look at the executive female who has her career in order. The corporate ladder was a breeze for her and everything she owns is from the top of the line. To see her is a dream for a man. In both cases, who knows what lies within? Are there regular doctor visits for treatments? Are there several prescriptions to prevent breakouts? To see their external appearance and the image of him or her, no one would be the wiser. Marriage is the only grounds for sexual intercourse, which will prevent exposure to STDs if both partners stay within the marriage and not explore the unknown.

The secular world wants to feel comfortable in the things they do; therefore, if those of us who worship Jesus Christ participate in the same secular things as the world, it will hinder their choice to live godly, and it will justify worldliness in their eye sight. Furthermore, they will publicly identify Christians as hypocrites. To some it makes no difference how they are viewed by others. They are worldly and proud of it. The only thing that they enjoy as much as worldly pleasures is to call-out Christians for participating in any sinful act. So, don't be fooled by those who wish to pull you down with deception or conning words. Smooth talkers are not always obvious, because they are sometimes extremely clever. Keep your guard up and be mindful of how you are approached for dating, job opportunities, and friendships. Their motives might not be known until they have gained your trust, possibly after you have grown to love him or her, which makes it harder to walk away.

The world is full of seducers both male and female who are ready to take advantage of anyone who will be taken in by them. Unbelievably, they like to entice the respected, innocent, low-keyed, and meek hearted individuals. Those who are in the clubs, who run the streets, or live life in the fast lane, are easy. They challenge themselves on those who are not so easy, so be aware. Your soul is the most valuable thing you have and your body is its dwelling place, so don't treat it like it is cheap. Protect it, take care of it, and keep it clean from spiritual and physical filth. Cover your body and respect it, because if you don't respect yourself, no one else will.

It's okay to be attractive and it's okay to be handsome. Exercise, eat healthy, and take care of your body, after all, it is the temple of God. Dress conservatively in neat apparel. Looking nice wearing daily and dressy attire is okay as long as it is not too tight or revealing. The phase, "Dressing sexy," has been used in many cases, but it implies that the individual has intentions to excite sexual desires. This is not the message we want to send out with our bodies. When others see us, we want them to see godliness, intellect, and class. Therefore, we should maintain moral standards in our behavior and appearances.

Recap:

This world we live in has a way of making wrong appear to be right. It presents bad things as good and good things bad. Worldliness makes the mind crave after sin and seek ways to obtain it. It has a way of forcing your imagination to fantasize about the very things that will eventually destroy you. Worldliness has no feelings or emotion just drive. The people that give in to worldliness know how to manipulate the minds of the weak and to feed off of them. If not careful, the strong minded can be drawn in as well because Satan is a master deceiver. For this reason, you must stay focused on the Lord. Prioritize your life by putting God first in everything that you do. You should focus on positive things in your life and not tune in to the negative things or your short comings. When you know that sex has a hold on you, you can't continue to do things that will naturally pull at you. Change your music, eliminate the sinful crowd, and walk away from movies pushing sexuality and lust if you truly want to make a change.

Maintain a prayerful life and keep God in your thoughts daily. Without Christ we can do nothing, but through Him, all things are possible. God will keep us if we truly want to be kept. Always remember to pray in faith. *James 1:6-8 says, But let him ask in faith, nothing wavering. For he that wavereth is like a wave of the sea driven with the wind and tossed. For let not that man think that he shall receive any thing of the Lord. A double minded man is unstable in all his ways (KJV).*

If we ask God to deliver us in faith, we can't say with our mouth, "Deliver me," but think in our minds, "I'm going to do it again." God knows the heart of every man; therefore, He knows the heart of the sincere man as well as the heart of the double minded. In other words, "We can't fool God." With this in mind, don't request forgiveness from God unless we are sincere about making a spiritual change. Instead, ask for deliverance from your strong holds.

Colossians 3:1-2 & 5&6 If ye then be risen with Christ, seek those things which are above, where Christ sitteth on the right hand of God. 2ⁿᵈ Set your affection on things above, not on things on the earth. 5ᵗʰ Mortify therefore your members which are upon the earth; fornication, uncleanness, inordinate affection, evil concupiscence, and covetousness, which is idolatry: 6ᵗʰ For which things' sake the wrath of God cometh on the children of disobedience: (KJV)

The Foundation Of Christinity

1 Corinthians 3:11 For other foundation can no man lay than that is laid, which is Jesus Christ. (KJV)

Jesus is the Son of God whose beginning wasn't as God's Son, but the living Word of God. *John 1:1 In the beginning was the Word and the Word was with God and the Word was God. (KJV)* He became the Son of God when He took on flesh as He was planted in the womb of a virgin called, Mary, for the purpose of sacrificing His life for the sins of man. God himself took off His glory just for the sake of man. *John 1:14 And the Word was made flesh, and dwelt among us, (and we beheld his glory, the glory as of the only begotten of the Father,) full of grace and truth. (KJV)*

He was born in a stable with the animals and laid in a manger. Coming not in luxury, but as the least as man would consider. Although we don't know the actual date of His birth, we recognized December 25th, a day we call Christmas, to acknowledge His birth. (Those who spell

Christmas as, "Xmas," fail to realize the significance of that day for they removed the root of the word, which is where it gets its meaning).

Jesus lived on earth as a natural man for he endured hunger, sadness, anger, and temptation. His journey on earth was a pattern set for man to follow to obtain patience, self control, love, etc. When His time was completed on earth, He allowed Himself to be captured and crucified on the cross. He died and His body remained in the grave for three days, but He rose on the morning of the third day with all power in His hands. This is the foundation of the saints: the death, burial, and resurrection of Jesus Christ. *Phililppians 2:9-11 Wherefore God also hath highly exalted him, and given him a name which is above every name: That at the name of Jesus every knee should bow, of things in heaven, and things in earth, and things under the earth; And that every tongue should confess that Jesus Christ is Lord, to the glory of God the Father. (KJV)*

Jesus didn't have to die for us, but He did. Because of his sacrifice no man can enter into the kingdom of heaven except they go through Him. *John 14:6 Jesus saith unto him, I am the way, the truth, and the life: no man cometh unto the Father, but by me. (KJV)*

After His resurrection, He ascended into heaven and is now seated at the right hand of His Father in heaven. Although He left, He sent us a comforter, which is the

Holy Spirit. This is the spirit of God. God the Father, God the Son, and God the Holy Spirit is the trinity. Therefore, Christians pray to God by way of the Holy Spirit through Jesus Christ.

Jesus has done wonderful things for us not only to give us hope, but we now have power through Him to overcome the situations we face in this world. The Spirit of God lives in us to lead, guide, and direct our decisions and choices on a daily basis. The Holy Spirit also gives us strength to stand on godliness. God does not force us to be saved, but His Spirit is there if we make the choice to give our life to Him. Christianity is a freedom of choice not the burden of force. Live by Him in this temporary life to be with Him in eternal life or live for the world led by Satan and spend eternity in the lake of fire with him. Turn away from worldliness and confess hope in Christ if you have not made Him your personal savior. *Romans 10:9 That if thou shalt confess with thy mouth the Lord Jesus, and shalt believe in thine heart that God hath raised him from the dead, thou shalt be saved (KJV).*

Mark 8:34 …Whosoever will come after me, let him deny himself, and take up his cross, and follow me (KJV).

On your quest for a spiritual life be mindful of false teachers and preachers who only teach on prosperity. Study the Bible for yourself with help from your parents or a true spiritual leader who teaches against sin and whose sole message is based on the heavenly Father who has laid the foundation on the death, burial, and resurrection of His Son Jesus Christ.

Read the book of Romans to help strengthen your Christian walk.

"Diagnosis Vaginismus"

Vaginismus (văj″ĭn-ĭz′mŭs) is a medical condition caused by a traumatic incident involving a sexual encounter. It's a muscle spasm that causes the vagina to close which makes penetration extremely difficult. Some patients have to undergo anesthesia to handle the pressures of an annual exam. Some people diagnosed with Vaginismus are victims of rape or some other type of sexual abuse as defined by Wikipedia encyclopedia.

Often times, date rape and incest go unreported. As a result, sometimes you and/or others have to deal with the mental distress and physical pain of Vaginismus. Therapy is necessary to overcome this condition. Although Vaginismus is not a common medical condition, it has been reported in a small number of women in the United States according to Medline Plus, a service of the U.S. National Library of Medicine and the National Institutes of Health.

The purpose of this informative medical condition is to make young girls aware of the different illnesses that could become a part of their lives if they are not careful.

Be mindful of the guys you date and never let your guard down while on a date.

The following fictional story is an example of why date rape may go unreported and the end result.

"Date Rape"

Kristi was a junior in a well known high school where she maintained good grades and participated in several after school extra curricular activities. She was popular and well known for her Christian way of living. As anyone else, she has faltered and given in to her boyfriend, Steve, in a few sexual encounters. Steve was a senior and the captain of the basketball team, but he also played football. As you can see, he was an all-around athletic guy who could play many different sports. He also maintained good grades. As a matter of fact, he received a full scholarship in sports as well as academics. In addition, he was approved for scholarships at several other prestigious colleges. Although Steve was a fairly nice guy, he couldn't understand the full concept of Christianity. He believed that there was a God, but he couldn't get with what some called, "the Jesus thing."

Kristi and Steve both had godly parents who taught them about the death, burial, and resurrection of Jesus Christ. Steve just had a personal problem believing the whole truth. Kristi actually gave a fifteen minute talk during study hall to talk with other students about the Bible with the principal's approval. This is why she was also well known by the faculty in addition to being studious.

One night while on a date, Steve continuously reminded Kristi of their love for each other and how good they were together. She melted inside and accepted his comments by sealing it with a kiss. One thing led to the next and before she knew it, they were both half undressed. She stopped him by pushing her body away from his. "What's wrong?" Steve asked. "Well, maybe we shouldn't do this," she answered in a soft timid voice. "Why not, we've had sex before? Is it that time of the month?" "No," she replied. "I've been reading and, well, fornication is wrong." "You are kidding right, I mean, this is a joke?" "No," Kristi stated. Steve sat back on the sofa and continued to murmur comments to himself. Kristi looked at him and sensitively asked, "Are you mad at me?" "Mad! No, I'm not mad," he replied. "I just can't understand why you would do this to me, knowing how much I love you and enjoy being with you like this," he said in a pleading voice. "I'm sorry, but after I read the Bible, I talked to two adults who assured me that it's wrong," she explained. "Adults talked to you about sex and now our life together is over?" "No," she answered. "Our life together isn't over, just the sexual part of it." Steve became very quiet and didn't say a word for about ten minutes. After the first five minutes past, Kristi turned off the radio and turned on the television. After five minutes of television, Steve nicely turned the radio back on then turned off the television. Kristi wondered to herself what he was thinking. Before she could get his name completely out, he kissed her passionately and told her how much he loved her. She returned the kiss, but he proceeded to go further. She began to push him away, but he resisted her rejection and pursued the sexual encounter. Her parents were upstairs, and he was so forceful that she didn't make much noise. Not to mention she was mentally in disbelief that she was being raped by her boyfriend. Nevertheless, he was much stronger than she was, and his mouth pressed so tightly against hers, she couldn't scream. After he raped her, he left and she couldn't move. Her dad came down the stairs around eleven o'clock, but Steve was gone and she covered herself with a throw blanket and shouted to her dad, "Steve has been gone for a while. I'm just going to finish watching this movie." "But honey, the television isn't on," her dad said in wonder. "Oh, I fell asleep…sleep mode must have been on to shut off the TV," she said. "Okay? Just don't stay up too late," he said as he walked back up stairs.

She turned on the television and laid there in tears not knowing what to think or how to think.

She woke up Saturday morning still in disbelief. All she could think about was how awful Monday morning was going to be when she would have to face everyone, including Steve. On that faithful morning the first person she saw was Steve with a cheerleader in his arms. Kristi was crushed. Later that day, the two of them ran into each other in the hallway. He told her that he still loved her, but life goes on. He tried to justify his actions by telling her that what happened Friday night was the two of them telling one another good-bye. He continued with words of encouragement about her future. She could not believe what she was hearing. In a burst of anger with tears rolling down her face she said, "You raped me." "How can you say that?" Steve replied, "Sure it was different from our other times together, but it was still us expressing our love towards each other." "What!" cried Kristi? "Why the new girl-friend if it was love Steve, uh, why? Explain that since you have all the answers," Kristi said in anger, but with a sad voice. Steve replied, "Sex was a part of our relationship and when you took that away, you took away fifty percent of the relationship. So, we were bound to lose interest in each other once you eliminated the biggest part of us. I'm making it easy for the both of us, so that we won't have to go through anymore misunderstood evenings." He walked away from her, and they never spoke to each other again.

Several years later, Kristi was pursuing her education in college. She talked with different guys as friends, but hadn't dated since her last relationship with Steve. She was living a pretty normal life for a twenty-one year old. She concentrated on her studies, continued to read her Bible, hung-out with friends, and maintained her good reputation.

One day she realized that she was having problems with her menstrual cycle. So, she made an appointment with a gynecologist (GYN). During her visit she didn't quite know what to expect. As her doctor began the exam, Kristi began to feel uncomfortable. Once the actual exam began, she was screaming out of control. Her doctor immediately ceased from finishing the exam. Kristi got dressed and stormed out of the examination room and continued to her dorm. Her doctor tried to reach her, but she would not return her phone calls. One day Kristi's girlfriend, Courtney, answered her phone; it was Kristi's doctor. Courtney tried to convince Kristi to go back to her doctor and complete the exam. After two months, Kristi finally decided to go back for the exam, but she would only go if Courtney went with her. On the day of the exam, Kristi was nervous, but Courtney held her hand the entire time. During the examination, Kristi experienced the trauma, only this time she didn't leave, but her doctor discontinued the exam. "What's wrong with me?" Kristi asked in tears. Her doctor instructed Kristi to get dressed and wait in her office to discuss what had just happened. The doctor first asked Kristi if she had any form of sexual abuse. Kristi hesitated, then she answered, "When I was in the eleventh grade, I was raped by my boyfriend. I never told anyone because we were sexually involved before that night, so I didn't think anyone would believe that it was rape. Furthermore, I didn't want to hurt my parents by taking them through court on a case that I was destined to lose." Courtney squeezed Kristi's hand and told her how sorry she was that such a thing had happened. The doctor sympathized with her as well. She then referred her to a Christian counselor who was a member of her church. She explained a condition called "Vaginismus" and how the vaginal muscles contracts and reacts to contact, mostly during sexual intercourse or pelvic exams. She also explained that this condition does not have to prevent her from having a sexual relationship with her future husband nor having children. A person with this condition can make a complete recovery with counseling and other techniques introduced by the counselor and/or a gynecologist.

Kristi sought the counselor and along with prayer, made a complete recovery. It took time, but faith in God and persistence were the key. She graduated from college with honors, obtained a respectable job, met a Christian man, married, and lived a fulfilled life.

Encouragement: This condition exists in females young and old, but it is not untreatable. This story is fiction, but the circumstances and the diagnosis could become a reality. If you are a victim, there is help and you can overcome it. Don't allow it to control you nor your future marriage. God has power to handle any situation and he understands all circumstances.

Scriptures For Encouragement and Guidance:

I Corinthians 10:13 There hath no temptation taken you but such as is common to man: but God is faithful, who will not suffer you to be tempted above that ye are able; but will with the temptation also make a way to escape, that ye may be able to bear it. (KJV)

Phililppians 4:13 I can do all things through Christ which strengtheneth me. (KJV)

James 4:10 Humble yourselves in the sight of the Lord, and he shall lift you up. (KJV)

Romans 8:31 What shall we then say to these things? If God be for us, who can be against us? (KJV)

1 Peter 5:7 Casting all your care upon him; for he careth for you. (KJV)

II Timothy 4:18 And the Lord shall deliver me from every evil work, and will preserve me unto his heavenly kingdom: to whom be glory for ever and ever. Amen (KJV)

James 1:12 Blessed is the man that endureth temptation: for when he is tried, he shall receive the crown of life, which the Lord hath promised to them that love him. (KJV)

A Message for Believers:

Sometimes bad decisions can give others the wrong impression of who you really are. Living with these choices can sometime give a false perception that can cause depression. In spite of what you have done always remember that God loves you and nothing can separate you from His love.

(Read these verses for encouragement).

Romans 8:35-39 Who shall separate us from the love of Christ? Shall tribulation, or distress, or persecution, or famine, or nakedness, or peril, or sword? As it is written, For thy sake we are killed all the day long; we are accounted as sheep for the slaughter. Nay, in all these things we are more than conquerors through him that loved us. For I am persuaded, that neither death, nor life, nor angels, nor principalities, nor powers, nor things present, nor things to come, Nor height, nor depth, nor any other creature, shall be able to separate us from the love of God, which is in Christ Jesus our Lord. (KJV)

A Verse to Make Your Personal Prayer:

Ephesians 1:17 That the God of our Lord Jesus, the Father of glory, may give unto you the spirit of wisdom and revelation in the knowledge of him: (KJV)

(Dear God, the God of our Lord Jesus, the Father of glory. Give me the spirit of wisdom and revelation in the knowledge of you).

The information in the following section is provided by:

CENTERS FOR DISEASE CONTROL

(CDC)

Sexually Transmitted Diseases

CHANCROID

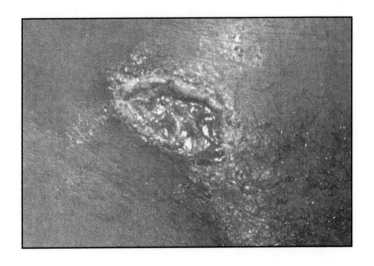

This photograph depicts a necrotic bubo in the inguinal region resulting from chancroid.

The first sign of infection is usually the appearance of one or more sores, or raised bumps on the genital organs. Sores are surrounded by a narrow red border.

It soon becomes filled with pus, and eventually ruptures, leaving a painful open wound.

A treatable bacterial infection that causes painful sores. Chancroid is a highly contagious yet curable sexually transmitted disease (STD) caused by the bacteria Haemophilus Ducreyi [hum-AH-fill-us DOO-cray]. Chancroid causes ulcers, usually of the genitals.

CHLAMYDIA

Chlamydia is a common sexually transmitted disease (STD) caused by the bacterium, Chlamydia trachomatis. Even though symptoms of chlamydia are usually mild or absent, serious complications that cause irreversible damage, including infertility and damage to a woman's reproductive organs can occur "silently" before a woman ever recognizes a problem. Chlamydia also can cause discharge from the penis of an infected man.

CRABS

Also known as pediculosis pubis, crabs are parasites or bugs that live on the pubic hair in the genital area

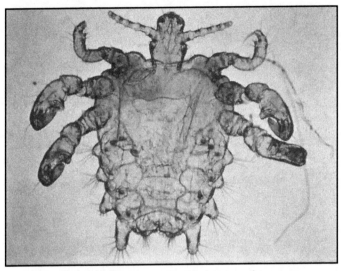

This is an enlargement of a Phthirus pubis, or more commonly known as the pubic or crab louse.

Normally, Phthirus pubis is transmitted from person to person through direct sexual contact, and thereafter, infest the widely spaced pubic hair region in adults, and the eye lashes in affected children.

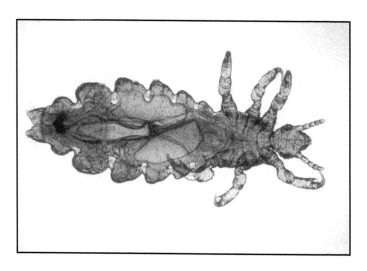

This image depicts a dorsal view of a female head louse, Pediculus humanus var. capitis.

These insects use their hook-like appendages to grasp unto the hair shafts of their hosts in body regions unique to its species, i.e. the head louse infests the head region of its host, while the pubic louse infests its host's pubic region.

What are pubic lice?

Also called "crabs," pubic lice are parasitic insects found in the genital area of humans. Infection is common and found worldwide.

How did I get pubic lice?

Pubic lice are usually spread through sexual contact. Rarely, infestation can be spread through contact with an infested person's bed linens, towels, or clothes. A common misunderstanding is that infestation can be spread by sitting on a toilet seat. This isn't likely, since lice cannot live long away from a warm human body. Also, lice do not have feet designed to walk or hold onto smooth surfaces such as toilet seats.

Infection in a young child or teenager may indicate sexual activity or sexual abuse.

Where are pubic lice found?

Pubic lice are generally found in the genital area on pubic hair; but may occasionally be found on other coarse body hair, such as hair on the legs, armpits, mustache, beard, eyebrows, or eyelashes. Infestations of young children are usually on the eyebrows or eyelashes. Lice found on the head are not pubic lice; they are head lice.

Animals do not get or spread pubic lice.

Signs and symptoms of pubic lice include

- Itching in the genital area
- Visible nits (lice eggs) or crawling lice

What do pubic lice look like?

There are three stages in the life of a pubic louse: the nit, the nymph, and the adult.

Nit: Nits are pubic lice eggs. They are hard to see and are found firmly attached to the hair shaft.

They are about the size of the mark at the end of this arrow . They are oval and usually yellow to white. Nits take about 1 week to hatch.

Nymph: The nit hatches into a baby louse called a nymph. It looks like an adult pubic louse, but it is smaller. Nymphs mature into adults about 7 days after hatching. To live, the nymph must feed on blood.

Adult: The adult pubic louse is about the size of this circle and resembles a miniature crab when viewed through a strong magnifying glass. Pubic lice have six legs, but their two front legs are very large and look like the pincher claws of a crab; this is how they got the nickname "crabs." Pubic lice are tan to grayish-white in color. Females lay nits and are usually larger than males. To live, adult lice must feed on blood. If the louse falls off a person, it dies within 1-2 days.

GONORRHEA

A treatable bacterial infection of the penis, vagina or anus that causes pain, or burning feeling as well as a pus-like discharge. Also known as "the clap".

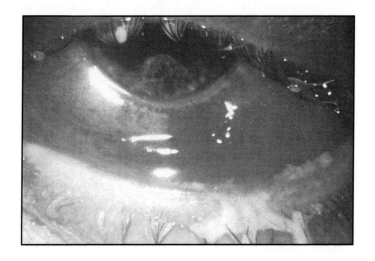

This case of gonorrheal conjunctivitis resulted in partial blindness due to the spread of N. gonorrhoeae bacteria.

Gonococci cause both localized infections, usually in the genital tract, and disseminated infections with seeding of various organs. Diagnosis of localized infections depends on Gram-staining, and culture of the discharge.

WHAT IS GONORRHEA?

Gonorrhea is a sexually transmitted disease (STD). Gonorrhea is caused by Neisseria gonorrhoeae, a bacterium that can grow and multiply easily in the warm, moist areas of the reproductive tract, including the cervix (opening to the womb), uterus (womb), and fallopian tubes (egg canals) in women, and in the urethra (urine canal) in women and men. The bacterium can also grow in the mouth, throat, eyes, and anus.

HOW DO PEOPLE GET GONORRHEA?

Gonorrhea is spread through contact with the penis, vagina, mouth, or anus. Ejaculation does not have to occur for gonorrhea to be transmitted or acquired. Gonorrhea can also be spread from mother to baby during delivery.

People who have had gonorrhea and received treatment may get infected again if they have sexual contact with a person infected with gonorrhea.

WHAT ARE THE SIGNS AND SYMPTOMS OF GONORRHEA?

Although many men with gonorrhea may have no symptoms at all, some men have some signs or symptoms that appear two to five days after infection; symptoms can take as long as 30 days to appear. Symptoms and signs include a burning sensation when urinating, or a white, yellow, or green discharge from the penis. Sometimes men with gonorrhea get painful or swollen testicles.

In women, the symptoms of gonorrhea are often mild, but most women who are infected have no symptoms. Even when a woman has symptoms, they can be so non-specific as to be mistaken for a bladder or vaginal infection. The initial symptoms and signs in women include a painful or burning sensation when urinating, increased vaginal discharge, or vaginal bleeding between periods. Women with gonorrhea are at risk of developing serious complications from the infection, regardless of the presence or severity of symptoms.

Symptoms of rectal infection in both men and women may include discharge, anal itching, soreness, bleeding, or painful bowel movements. Rectal infection also may cause no symptoms. Infections in the throat may cause a sore throat but usually causes no symptoms.

WHAT ARE THE COMPLICATIONS OF GONORRHEA?

Untreated gonorrhea can cause serious and permanent health problems in both women and men.

In women, gonorrhea is a common cause of pelvic inflammatory disease (PID). About one million women each year in the United States develop PID. Women with PID do not necessarily have symptoms. When symptoms are present, they can be very severe and can include abdominal pain and fever. PID can lead to internal abscesses (pus-filled "pockets" that are hard to cure) and long-lasting, chronic pelvic pain. PID can damage the fallopian tubes enough to cause infertility or increase the risk of ectopic pregnancy. Ectopic pregnancy is a life-threatening condition in which a fertilized egg grows outside the uterus, usually in a fallopian tube.

In men, gonorrhea can cause epididymitis, a painful condition of the testicles that can lead to infertility if left untreated.

Gonorrhea can spread to the blood or joints. This condition can be life threatening. In addition, people with gonorrhea can more easily contract HIV, the virus that causes AIDS. HIV-infected people with gonorrhea are more likely to transmit HIV to someone else.

HOW DOES GONORRHEA AFFECT A PREGNANT WOMAN AND HER BABY?

If a pregnant woman has gonorrhea, she may give the infection to her baby as the baby passes through the birth canal during delivery. This can cause blindness, joint infection, or a life-threatening blood infection in the baby. Treatment of gonorrhea as soon as it is detected in pregnant women will reduce the risk of these complications. Pregnant women should consult a health care provider for appropriate examination,

HEPATITIS B

A disease that affects the liver. There are more than four types. A and B are the most common.

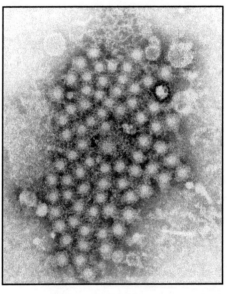

This transmission electron micrograph (TEM) revealed numerous hepatitis virions, of an unknown strain of the organism. In the United States, viral hepatitis is an important public health problem because it causes serious illness, it affects millions, and it has a close connection with HIV. There are five identified types of viral hepatitis and each one is caused by a different virus. In the United States, hepatitis A, hepatitis B and hepatitis C are the most common types.

Hepatitis A is a liver disease caused by the hepatitis A virus (HAV), and can affect anyone. In the U. S., hepatitis A occurs in situations ranging from isolated cases, to widespread epidemics.

Hepatitis B is a serious disease caused by a virus that attacks the liver. Known as hepatitis B virus (HBV), it can cause lifelong infection, cirrhosis (scarring) of the liver, liver cancer, liver failure, and death.

Hepatitis C is a liver disease caused by the hepatitis C virus (HCV), which is found in the blood of persons who have the disease. HCV is spread by contact with the blood of an infected person.

Hepatitis D is a liver disease caused by the hepatitis D virus (HDV), a defective virus that needs the HBV virus to exist. HDV is found in the blood of persons infected with the virus.

Hepatitis E is a liver disease caused by the hepatitis E virus (HEV), transmitted in much the same way as hepatitis A virus. Hepatitis E, however, does not occur often in the United States.

Hepatitis A is a liver disease caused by the hepatitis A virus. Hepatitis A can affect anyone. In the United States, hepatitis A can occur in situations ranging from isolated cases of disease to widespread epidemics.

Good personal hygiene and proper sanitation can help prevent hepatitis A. Vaccines are also available for long-term prevention of hepatitis A virus infection in persons 12 months of age and older. Immune globulin is available for short-term prevention of hepatitis A virus infection in individuals of all ages.

Hepatitis B is a serious disease caused by a virus that attacks the liver. The virus, which is called hepatitis B virus (HBV), can cause lifelong infection, cirrhosis (scarring) of the liver, liver cancer, liver failure, and death.

Hepatitis B vaccine is available for all age groups to prevent hepatitis B virus infection.

HERPES

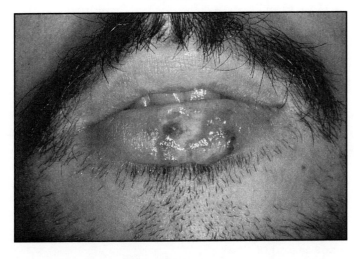

Photo Credit: Sol Silverman, Jr., D.D.S.
This HIV-positive patient was exhibiting a chronic
mucocutaneous herpes lesion for one month in duration.

Herpes simplex virus type1 usually is the cause for oral lesions sometimes referred to as "cold sores", "fever blisters" or more technically known as "recurrent herpes labialis".

Genital herpes is a recurrent skin condition that can cause skin irritations in the genital region (anus, vagina, penis).

WHAT IS GENITAL HERPES?

Genital herpes is a sexually transmitted disease (STD) caused by the herpes simplex viruses type 1 (HSV-1) and type 2 (HSV-2). Most genital herpes is caused by HSV-2. Most individuals have no or only minimal signs or symptoms from HSV-1 or HSV-2 infection. When signs do occur, they typically appear as one or more blisters on or around the genitals or rectum. The blisters break, leaving tender ulcers (sores) that may take two to four weeks to heal the first time they occur. Typically, another outbreak can appear weeks or months after the first, but it almost always is less severe and shorter than the first outbreak. Although the infection can stay in the body indefinitely, the number of outbreaks tends to decrease over a period of years.

HOW DO PEOPLE GET GENITAL HERPES?

HSV-1 and HSV-2 can be found in and released from the sores that the viruses cause, but they also are released between outbreaks from skin that does not appear to be broken or to have a sore. Generally, a person can only get HSV-2 infection during sexual contact with someone who has a genital HSV-2 infection. Transmission can occur from an infected partner who does not have a visible sore and may not know that he or she is infected.

HSV-1 can cause genital herpes, but it more commonly causes infections of the mouth and lips, so-called "fever blisters." HSV-1 infection of the genitals can be caused by oral-genital or genital-genital contact with a person who has HSV-1 infection. Genital HSV-1 outbreaks recur less regularly than genital HSV-2 outbreaks.

WHAT ARE THE SIGNS AND SYMPTOMS OF GENITAL HERPES?

Most people infected with HSV-2 are not aware of their infection. However, if signs and symptoms occur during the first outbreak, they can be quite pronounced. The first outbreak usually occurs within two weeks after the virus is transmitted, and the sores typically heal within two to four weeks. Other signs and symptoms during the primary episode may include a second crop of sores, and flu-like symptoms, including fever and swollen glands.

However, most individuals with HSV-2 infection may never have sores, or they may have very mild signs that they do not even notice or that they mistake for insect bites or another skin condition.

Most people diagnosed with a first episode of genital herpes can expect to have several (typically four or five) outbreaks (symptomatic recurrences) within a year. Over time these recurrences usually decrease in frequency.

WHAT ARE THE COMPLICATIONS OF GENITAL HERPES?

Genital herpes can cause recurrent painful genital sores in many adults, and herpes infection can be severe in people with suppressed immune systems. Regardless of severity of symptoms, genital herpes frequently causes psychological distress in people who know they are infected.

In addition, genital HSV can cause potentially fatal infections in babies. It is important that women avoid contracting herpes during pregnancy because a first episode during pregnancy causes a greater risk of transmission to the baby. If a woman has active genital herpes at delivery, a cesarean delivery is usually performed. Fortunately, infection of a baby from a woman with herpes infection is rare.

Herpes may play a role in the spread of HIV, the virus that causes AIDS. Herpes can make people more susceptible to HIV infection, and it can make HIV-infected individuals more infectious.

IS THERE A TREATMENT FOR HERPES?

There is no treatment that can cure herpes, but antiviral medications can shorten and prevent outbreaks during the period of time the person takes the medication. In addition, daily suppressive therapy for symptomatic herpes can reduce transmission to partners.

HUMAN PAPILLOMAVIRUS/GENITAL WARTS

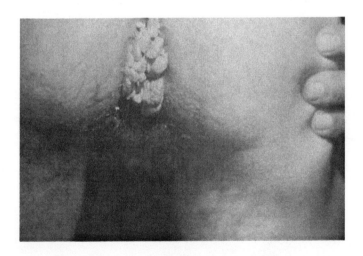

This male patient presented with venereal warts in the anal region of the perineum.

Condylomata acuminata, or genital warts, is a sexually transmitted disease caused by the Human Papilloma Virus, (HPV), which manifests as bumps or warts on the genitalia, or within the perineal region.

Human papillomavirus (HPV) is a virus that affects the skin in the genital area, as well as a female's cervix. Depending on the type of HPV involved, symptoms can be in the form of wart-like growths, or abnormal cell changes. For additional information on HPV go to the CDC website for HPV.

WHAT IS GENITAL HPV INFECTION?

Genital HPV infection is a sexually transmitted disease (STD) that is caused by human papillomavirus (HPV). Human papillomavirus is the name of a group of viruses that includes more than 100 different strains or types. More than 30 of these viruses are sexually transmitted, and they can infect the genital area of men and women including the skin of the penis, vulva (area outside the vagina), or anus, and the linings of the vagina, cervix, or rectum. Most people who become infected with HPV will not have any symptoms and will clear the infection on their own.

Some of these viruses are called "high-risk" types, and may cause abnormal Pap tests. They may also lead to cancer of the cervix, vulva, vagina, anus, or penis.

Others are called "low-risk" types, and they may cause mild Pap test abnormalities or genital warts. Genital warts are single or multiple growths or bumps that appear in the genital area, and sometimes are cauliflower shaped.

HOW COMMON IS HPV?

Approximately 20 million people are currently infected with HPV. At least 50 percent of sexually active men and women acquire genital HPV infection at some point in their lives. By age 50, at least 80 percent of women will have acquired genital HPV infection. About 6.2 million Americans get a new genital HPV infection each year.

HOW DO PEOPLE GET GENITAL HPV INFECTIONS?

The types of HPV that infect the genital area are spread primarily through genital contact. Most HPV infections have no signs or symptoms; therefore, most infected persons are unaware they are infected, yet they can transmit the virus to a sex partner. Rarely, a pregnant woman can pass HPV to her baby during vaginal delivery. A baby that is exposed to HPV very rarely develops warts in the throat or voice box.

WHAT ARE THE SIGNS AND SYMPTOMS OF GENITAL HPV INFECTION?

Most people who have a genital HPV infection do not know they are infected. The virus lives in the skin or mucous membranes and usually causes no symptoms. Some people get visible genital warts, or have pre-cancerous changes in the cervix, vulva, anus, or penis. Very rarely, HPV infection results in anal or genital cancers.

Genital warts usually appear as soft, moist, pink, or flesh-colored swellings, usually in the genital area. They can be raised or flat, single or multiple, small or large, and sometimes cauliflower shaped. They can appear on the vulva, in or around the vagina or anus, on the cervix, and on the penis, scrotum, groin, or thigh. After sexual contact with an infected person, warts may appear within weeks or months, or not at all.

Genital warts are diagnosed by visual inspection. Visible genital warts can be removed by medications the patient applies, or by treatments performed by a health care provider. Some individuals choose to forego treatment to see if the warts will disappear on their own. No treatment regimen for genital warts is better than another, and no one treatment regimen is ideal for all cases.

HOW IS GENITAL HPV INFECTED DIAGNOSED?

Most women are diagnosed with HPV on the basis of abnormal Pap tests. A Pap test is the primary cancer-screening tool for cervical cancer or pre-cancerous changes in the cervix, many of which are related to HPV. Also, a specific test is available to detect HPV DNA in women. The test may be used in women with mild Pap test abnormalities, or in women >30 years of age at the time of Pap testing. The results of HPV DNA testing can help health care providers decide if further tests or treatment are necessary.

No HPV tests are available for men.

IS THERE A CURE FOR HPV?

There is no "cure" for HPV infection, although in most women the infection goes away on its own. The treatments provided are directed to the changes in the skin or mucous membrane caused by HPV infection, such as warts and pre-cancerous changes in the cervix.

WHAT IS THE CONNECTION BETWEEN HPV INFECTION AND CERVICA CANCER?

All types of HPV can cause mild Pap test abnormalities which do not have serious consequences. Approximately 10 of the 30 identified genital HPV types can lead, in rare cases, to development of cervical cancer. Research has shown that for most women (90 percent), cervical HPV infection becomes undetectable within two years. Although only a small proportion of women have persistent infection, persistent infection with "high-risk" types of HPV is the main risk factor for cervical cancer.

A Pap test can detect pre-cancerous and cancerous cells on the cervix. Regular Pap testing and careful medical follow-up, with treatment if necessary, can help ensure that pre-cancerous changes in the cervix caused by HPV infection do not develop into life threatening cervical cancer. The Pap test used in U.S. cervical cancer screening programs is responsible for greatly reducing deaths from cervical cancer. For 2004, the American Cancer Society estimates that about 10,520 women will develop invasive cervical cancer and about 3,900 women will die from this disease. Most women who develop invasive cervical cancer have not had regular cervical cancer screening.

MOLLUSCUM CONTAGIOSUM

What is molluscum contagiosum?

A skin disease caused by the molluscum contagiosum virus (MCV) usually causing one or more small lesions/bumps. MCV is generally a benign infection and symptoms may self-resolve. MCV was once a disease primarily of children, but it has evolved to become a sexually transmitted disease in adults. It is believed to be a member of the pox virus family.

How is it transmitted?

- Molluscum contagiosum may be sexually transmitted by skin-to-skin contact (does not have to be mucous membranes) and/or lesions. Transmission through sexual contact is the most common form of transmission for adults.

- MCV may be transmitted from inanimate objects such as towels and clothing that come in contact with the lesions. MCV transmission has been associated with swimming pools and sharing baths with an infected person.

- MCV also may be transmitted by autoinoculation, such as touching a lesion and touching another part of the body. To stop from further spreading the infection, do not shave over or close to areas that are visibly infected.

What is the incubation period?

The incubation period averages 2 to 3 months and may range from 1 week to 6 months.

How long are you infectious?

This is not known for certain, but researchers assume that if the virus is present it may be transmitted.

Symptoms

- Lesions are usually present on the thighs, buttocks, groin and lower abdomen of adults, and may occasionally appear on the external genital and anal region.

- Children typically develop lesions on the face, trunk, legs and arms.

- The lesions may begin as small bumps which can develop over a period of several weeks into larger sores/bumps. The lesions can be flesh colored, gray-white, yellow or pink. They can cause itching or tenderness in the area, but in most cases the lesions cause few problems.

Lesions can last from 2 weeks to 4 years -- the average is 2 years.

• People with AIDS or others with compromised immune systems may develop extensive outbreaks.

NONGONOCOCCAL URETHRITIS (NGU)

What is NGU?

NGU (NonGonococcal Urethritis) is an infection of the urethra caused by pathogens (germs) other than gonorrhea.

Several kinds of pathogens can cause NGU, including:

• *Chlamydia trachomatis*

• *Ureaplasma urealyticum*

• *Trichomonas vaginalis (rare)*

• *Herpes simplex virus (rare)*

• *Adenovirus*

• *Haemophilus vaginalis*

• *Mycoplasm genitalium*

NGU is most often caused by chlamydia, a common infection in men and women. The diagnosis of NGU is more commonly made in men than women, primarily due to anatomical differences.

How is it transmitted?

<u>Sexual:</u>

Most germs that cause NGU can be passed during sex (vaginal, anal or oral) that involves direct mucous membrane contact with an infected person. These germs can be passed even if the penis or tongue does not go all the way into the vagina, mouth or rectum, and even if body fluids are not exchanged.

<u>Nonsexual:</u>

- Urinary tract infections.
- An inflamed prostate gland due to bacteria (bacterial prostatitis).
- A narrowing or closing of the tube in the penis (urethral stricture).
- A tightening of the foreskin so that it cannot be pulled back from the head of the penis (phimosa).

- The result of a process such as inserting a tube into the penis (catheterization).

Perinatal:

During birth, infants maybe exposed to the germs causing NGU in passage through the birth canal. This may cause the baby to have infections in the:

- eyes (conjunctivitis)
- ears
- lungs (pneumonia)

Symptoms

Men (urethral infection):

- Discharge from the penis
- Burning or pain when urinating (peeing)
- Itching, irritation, or tenderness
- Underwear stain

Women (vaginal/urethral infection):

The germs that cause NGU in men might cause other infections in women. These might include vaginitis or mucopurulent cervicitis (MPC). Women may also be asymptomatic (have no symptoms). Symptoms of NGU in women can include:

- Discharge from the vagina

- Burning or pain when urinating (peeing)

- Abdominal pain or abnormal vaginal bleeding may be an indication that the infection has progressed to Pelvic inflammatory Disease (PID)

Anal or Oral Infections Anal infection may result in: - Rectal itching - Discharge or pain on defecation Oral infection may occur. Most (90 percent) are asymptomatic, but some people might have a sore throat.

What does it mean for my health?

Left untreated, the germs that cause NGU-especially chlamydia-can lead to:

Men:

- Epididymitis (inflammation of the epididymis, the elongated, cordlike structure along the posterior border of the testes) which can lead to infertility if left untreated.

- Reiter's syndrome (arthritis)

- Conjunctivitis

- Skin lesions

- Discharge

<u>Women:</u>

- Pelvic Inflammatory Disease (PID) which can result in ectopic (tubal) pregnancy.

- Recurrent PID may lead to infertility.

- Chronic pelvic pain

- Urethritis

- Vaginitis

- Mucopurulent cervicitis (MPC)

- Spontaneous abortion (miscarriage)

<u>Men or Women:</u>

- Infections caused by anal sex might lead to severe proctitis (inflamed rectum).

<u>Infants:</u>

Exposure to the germs causing NGU during passage through the birth canal may result in infants having:

- Conjunctivitis (If left untreated, this may lead to blindness.)

- Pneumonia

PELVIS INFLAMMATORY DISEASE (PID)

WHAT IS PID?

Pelvic inflammatory disease (PID) is a general term that refers to infection of the uterus (womb), fallopian tubes (tubes that carry eggs from the ovaries to the uterus) and other reproductive organs. It is a common and serious complication of some sexually transmitted diseases (STDs), especially chlamydia and gonorrhea. PID can damage the fallopian tubes and tissues in and near the uterus and ovaries. Untreated PID can lead to serious consequences including infertility, ectopic pregnancy (a pregnancy in the fallopian tube or elsewhere outside of the womb), abscess formation, and chronic pelvic pain.

HOW COMMON IS PID?

Each year in the United States, it is estimated that more than 1 million women experience an episode of acute PID. More than 100,000 women become infertile each year as a result of PID, and a large proportion of the ectopic pregnancies occurring every year are due to the consequences of PID. Annually more than 150 women die from PID or its complications.

HOW DO WOMEN GET PID?

PID occurs when bacteria move upward from a woman's vagina or cervix (opening to the uterus) into her reproductive organs. Many different organisms can cause PID, but many cases are associated with gonorrhea and chlamydia, two very common bacterial STDs. A prior episode of PID increases the risk of another episode because the reproductive organs may be damaged during the initial bout of infection.

Sexually active women in their childbearing years are most at risk, and those under age 25 are more likely to develop PID than those older than 25. This is because the cervix of teenage girls and young women is not fully matured, increasing their susceptibilty to the STDs that are linked to PID.

The more sex partners a woman has, the greater her risk of developing PID. Also, a woman whose partner has more than one sex partner is at greater risk of developing PID, because of the potential for more exposure to infectious agents.

Women who douche may have a higher risk of developing PID compared with women who do not douche. Research has shown that douching changes the vaginal flora (organisms that live in the vagina) in harmful ways, and can force bacteria into the upper reproductive organs from the vagina.

Women who have an intrauterine device (IUD) inserted may have a slightly increased risk of PID near the time of insertion compared with women using other contraceptives or no contraceptive at all. However, this risk is greatly reduced if a woman is tested and, if necessary, treated for STDs before an IUD is inserted.

WHAT ARE THE SIGNS AND SYMPTOMS OF PID?

Symptoms of PID vary from none to severe. When PID is caused by chlamydial infection, a woman may experience mild symptoms or no symptoms at all, while serious damage is being done to her reproductive organs. Because of vague symptoms, PID goes unrecognized by women and their health care providers about two thirds of the time. Women who have symptoms of PID most commonly have lower abdominal pain. Other signs and symptoms include fever, unusual vaginal discharge that may have a foul odor, painful intercourse, painful urination, irregular menstrual bleeding, and pain in the right upper abdomen (rare).

WHAT ARE THE COMPLICATIONS OF PID?

Prompt and appropriate treatment can help prevent complications of PID. Without treatment, PID can cause permanent damage to the female reproductive organs.

Infection-causing bacteria can silently invade the fallopian tubes, causing normal tissue to turn into scar tissue. This scar tissue blocks or interrupts the normal movement of eggs into the uterus. If the fallopian tubes are totally blocked by scar tissue, sperm cannot fertilize an egg, and the woman becomes infertile. Infertility also can occur if the fallopian tubes are partially blocked or even slightly damaged. About one in eight women with PID becomes infertile, and if a woman has multiple episodes of PID, her chances of becoming infertile increase.

In addition, a partially blocked or slightly damaged fallopian tube may cause a fertilized egg to remain in the fallopian tube. If this fertilized egg begins to grow in the tube as if it were in the uterus, it is called an ectopic pregnancy. As it grows, an ectopic pregnancy can rupture the fallopian tube causing severe pain, internal bleeding, and even death.

Scarring in the fallopian tubes and other pelvic structures can also cause chronic pelvic pain (pain that lasts for months or even years). Women with repeated episodes of PID are more likely to suffer infertility, ectopic pregnancy, or chronic pelvic pain.

HOW IS PID DIAGNOSED?

PID is difficult to diagnose because the symptoms are often subtle and mild. Many episodes of PID go undetected because the woman or her health care provider fails to recognize the implications of mild or nonspecific symptoms. Because there are no precise tests for PID, a diagnosis is usually based on clinical findings. If symptoms such as lower abdominal pain are present, a health care provider should perform a physical examination to determine the nature and location of the pain and chek for fever, abnormal vaginal or cervical discharge, and for evidence of gonorrheal or chlamydial infection. If the findings suggest PID, treatment is necessary.

WHAT IS THE TREATMENT FOR PID?

PID can be cured with several types of antibiotics. A health care provider will determine and prescribe the best therapy. However, antibiotic treatment does not reverse any damage that has already occurred to the reproductive organs. If a woman has pelvic pain and other symptoms of PID, it is critical that she seek care immediately. Prompt antibiotic treatment can prevent severe damage to reproductive organs. The longer a woman delays treatment for PID, the more likely she is to become infertile or to have a future ectopic pregnancy because of damage to the fallopian tubes.

Because of the difficulty in identifying organisms infecting the internal reproductive organs and because more than one organism may be responsible for an episode of PID, PID is usually treated with at least two antibiotics that are effective against a wide range of infectious agents. These antibiotics can be given by mouth or by injection. The symptoms may go away before the infection is cured. Even if symptoms go away, the woman should finish taking all of the prescribed medicine. This will help prevent the infection from returning. Women being treated for PID should be re-evaluated by their health care provider two to three days after starting treatment to be sure the antibiotics are working to cure the infection. In addition, a woman's sex partner(s) should be treated to decrease the risk of re-infection, even if the partner(s) has no symptoms. Although sex partners may have no symptoms, they may still be infected with the organisms that can cause PID.

Hospitalization to treat PID may be recommended if the woman (1) is severely ill (e.g., nausea, vomiting, and high fever); (2) is pregnant; (3) does not respond to or cannot take oral medication and needs intravenous antibiotics; or (4) has an abscess in the fallopian tube or ovary (tubo-ovarian abscess). If symptoms continue or if an abscess does not go away, surgery may be needed. Complications of PID, such as chronic pelvic pain and scarring are difficult to treat, but sometimes they improve with surgery

SCABIES

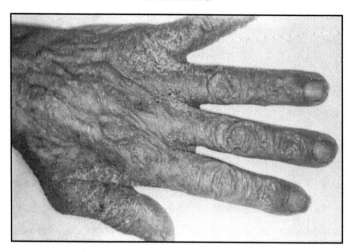

Photo Credit: Reed and Carnrich Pharmaceuticals.
This patient's hand reveals a scabies infestation of the mite
species Sarcoptes scabiei var. hominis.

The scabies rash manifests itself as pimple-like eruptions, especially within the webbing between the fingers, the skin folds on the wrist, elbow or knee, the penis, breast, and shoulder blades.

Scabies is an infestation of the skin with the microscopic mite Sarcoptes scabei. Infestation is common, found worldwide, and affects people of all races and social classes. Scabies spreads rapidly under crowded conditions where there is frequent skin-to-skin contact between people, such as in hospitals, institutions, child-care facilities, and nursing homes

What is scabies?

Scabies is an infestation of the skin with the microscopic mite Sarcoptes scabei. Infestation is common, found worldwide, and affects people of all races and social classes. Scabies spreads rapidly under crowded conditions where there is frequent skin-to-skin contact between people, such as in hospitals, institutions, child-care facilities, and nursing homes.

What are the signs and symptoms of scabies infestation?

- Pimple-like irritations, burrows or rash of the skin, especially the webbing between the fingers; the skin folds on the wrist, elbow, or knee; the penis, the breast, or shoulder blades.

- Intense itching, especially at night and over most of the body.

- Sores on the body caused by scratching. These sores can sometimes become infected with bacteria.

How did I get scabies?

By direct, prolonged, skin-to-skin contact with a person already infested with scabies. Contact must be prolonged (a quick handshake or hug will usually not spread infestation). Infestation is easily spread to sexual partners and household members. Infestation may also occur by sharing clothing, towels, and bedding.

Who is at risk for severe infestation?

People with weakened immune systems and the elderly are at risk for a more severe form of scabies, called Norwegian or crusted scabies.

How long will mites live?

Once away from the human body, mites do not survive more than 48-72 hours. When living on a person, an adult female mite can live up to a month.

Did my pet spread scabies to me?

No. Pets become infested with a different kind of scabies mite. If your pet is infested with scabies, (also called mange) and they have close contact with you, the mite can get under your skin and cause itching and skin irritation. However, the mite dies in a couple of days and does not reproduce. The mites may cause you to itch for several days, but you do not need to be treated with special medication to kill the mites. Until your pet is successfully treated, mites can continue to burrow into your skin and cause you to have symptoms.

How soon after infestation will symptoms begin?

For a person who has never been infested with scabies, symptoms may take 4-6 weeks to begin. For a person who has had scabies, symptoms appear within several days. You do not become immune to an infestation.

How is scabies infestation diagnosed?

Diagnosis is most commonly made by looking at the burrows or rash. A skin scraping may be taken to look for mites, eggs, or mite fecal matter to confirm the diagnosis. If a skin scraping or biopsy is taken and returns negative, it is possible that you may still be infested. Typically, there are fewer than 10 mites on the entire body of an infested person; this makes it easy for an infestation to be missed.

Can scabies be treated?

Yes. Several lotions are available to treat scabies. Always follow the directions provided by your physician or the directions on the package insert. Apply lotion to a clean body from the neck down to the toes and left overnight (8 hours). After 8 hours, take a bath or shower to wash off the lotion. Put on clean clothes. All clothes, bedding, and towels used by the infested person 2 days before treatment should be washed in hot water; dry in a hot dryer. A second treatment of the body with the same lotion may be necessary 7-10 days later. Pregnant women and children are often treated with milder scabies medications.

Who should be treated for scabies?

Anyone who is diagnosed with scabies, as well as his or her sexual partners and persons who have close, prolonged contact to the infested person should also be treated. If your health care provider has instructed family members to be treated, everyone should receive treatment at the same time to prevent reinfestation.

How soon after treatment will I feel better?

Itching may continue for 2-3 weeks, and does not mean that you are still infested. Your health care provider my prescribe additional medication to relieve itching if it is severe. No new burrows or rashes should appear 24-48 hours after effective treatment.

SYPHILIS

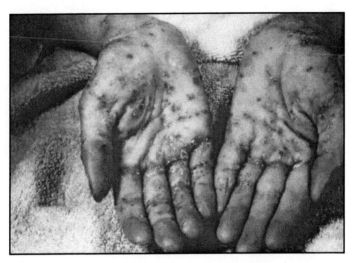

This photograph shows keratotic lesions on the palms of this patient's hands due to a secondary syphilitic infection.

Syphilis is a complex sexually transmitted disease (STD) caused by the bacterium Treponema pallidum. It has often been called "the great imitator" because so many of the signs and symptoms are indistinguishable from those of other diseases.

A treatable bacterial infection that can spread throughout the body and affect the heart, brain, nerves. Also known as "syph".

WHAT IS SYPHILIS?

Syphilis is a sexually transmitted disease (STD) caused by the bacterium Treponema pallidum. It has often been called "the great imitator" because so many of the signs and symptoms are indistinguishable from those of other diseases.

HOW COMMON IS SYPHILIS?

In the United States, health officials reported over 32,000 cases of syphilis in 2002, including 6,862 cases of primary and secondary (P&S) syphilis. In 2002, half of all P&S syphilis cases were reported from 16 counties and 1 city; and most P&S syphilis cases occurred in persons 20 to 39 years of age. The incidence of infectious syphilis was highest in women 20 to 24 years of age and in men 35 to 39 years of age. Reported cases of congenital syphilis in newborns decreased from 2001 to 2002, with 492 new cases reported in 2001 compared to 412 cases in 2002.

Between 2001 and 2002, the number of reported P & S syphilis cases increased 12.4 percent. Rates in women continued to decrease, and overall, the rate in men was 3.5 times that in women. This, in conjunction with reports of syphilis outbreaks in men who have sex with men (MSM), suggests that rates of syphilis in MSM are increasing.

HOW DO PEOPLE GET SYPHILIS?

Syphilis is passed from person to person through direct contact with a syphilis sore. Sores occur mainly on the external genitals, vagina, anus, or in the rectum. Sores also can occur on the lips and in the mouth. Transmission of the organism occurs during vaginal, anal, or oral sex. Pregnant women with the disease can pass it to the babies they are carrying. Syphilis cannot be spread through contact with toilet seats, doorknobs, swimming pools, hot tubs, bathtubs, shared clothing, or eating utensils.

WHAT ARE THE SIGNS AND SYMPTOMS IN ADULTS?

Many people infected with syphilis do not have any symptoms for years, yet remain at risk for late complications if they are not treated. Although transmission appears to occur from persons with sores who are in the primary or secondary stage, many of these sores are unrecognized. Thus, most transmission is from persons who are unaware of their infection.

Primary Stage

The primary stage of syphilis is usually marked by the appearance of a single sore (called a chancre), but there may be multiple sores. The time between infection with syphilis and the start of the first symptom can range from 10 to 90 days (average 21 days). The chancre is usually firm, round, small, and painless. It appears at the spot where syphilis entered the body. The chancre lasts 3 to 6 weeks, and it heals without treatment. However, if adequate treatment is not administered, the infection progresses to the secondary stage.

Secondary Stage

Skin rash and mucous membrane lesions characterize the secondary stage. This stage typically starts with the development of a rash on one or more areas of the body. The rash usually does not cause itching. Rashes associated with secondary syphilis can appear as the chancre is healing or several weeks after the chancre has healed. The characteristic rash of secondary syphilis may appear as rough, red, or reddish brown spots both on the palms of the hands and the bottoms of the feet. However, rashes with a different appearance may occur on other parts of the body, sometimes resembling rashes caused by other diseases. Sometimes rashes associated with secondary syphilis are so faint that they are not noticed. In addition to rashes, symptoms of secondary syphilis may include fever, swollen lymph glands, sore throat, patchy hair loss, headaches, weight loss, muscle aches, and fatigue. The signs and symptoms of secondary syphilis will resolve with or without treatment, but without treatment, the infection will progress to the latent and late stages of disease.

Late Stage

The latent (hidden) stage of syphilis begins when secondary symptoms disappear. Without treatment, the infected person will continue to have syphilis even though there are no signs or symptoms; infection remains in the body. In the late stages of syphilis, it may subsequently damage the internal organs, including the brain, nerves, eyes, heart, blood vessels, liver, bones, and joints. This internal damage may show up many years later. Signs and symptoms of the late stage of syphilis include difficulty coordinating muscle movements, paralysis, numbness, gradual blindness, and dementia. This damage may be serious enough to cause death.

HOW DOES SYPHILIS AFFECT A PREGNANT WOMAN AND HER BABY?

The syphilis bacterium can infect the baby of a woman during her pregnancy. Depending on how long a pregnant woman has been infected, she may have a high risk of having a stillbirth (a baby born dead) or of giving birth to a baby who dies shortly after birth. An infected baby may be born without signs or symptoms of disease. However, if not treated immediately, the baby may develop serious problems within a few weeks. Untreated babies may become developmentally delayed, have seizures, or die.

HOW IS SYPHILIS DIAGNOSED?

Some health care providers can diagnose syphilis by examining material from a chancre (infectious sore) using a special microscope called a dark-field microscope. If syphilis bacteria are present in the sore, they will show up when observed through the microscope.

A blood test is another way to determine whether someone has syphilis. Shortly after infection occurs, the body produces syphilis antibodies that can be detected by an accurate, safe, and inexpensive blood test. A low level of antibodies will stay in the blood for months or years even after the disease has been successfully treated. Because untreated syphilis in a pregnant woman can infect and possibly kill her developing baby, every pregnant woman should have a blood test for syphilis.

WHAT IS THE LINK BETWEEN SYPHILIS AND HIV?

Genital sores (chancres) caused by syphilis make it easier to transmit and acquire HIV infection sexually. There an estimated 2- to 5-fold increased risk of acquiring HIV infection when syphilis is present.

Ulcerative STDs that cause sores, ulcers, or breaks in the skin or mucous membranes, such as syphilis, disrupt barriers that provide protection against infections. The genital ulcers caused by syphilis can bleed easily, and when they come into contact with oral and rectal mucosa during sex, increase the infectiousness of and susceptibility to HIV. Having other STDs is also an important predictor for becoming HIV infected because STDs are a marker for behaviors associated with HIV transmission.

WHAT IS THE TREATMENT FOR SYPHILIS?

Syphilis is easy to cure in its early stages. A single intramuscular injection of penicillin, an antibiotic, will cure a person who has had syphilis for less than a year. Additional doses are needed to treat someone who has had syphilis for longer than a year. For people who are allergic to penicillin, other antibiotics are available to treat syphilis. There are no home remedies or over-the-counter drugs that will cure syphilis. Treatment will kill the syphilis bacterium and prevent further damage, but it will not repair damage already done.

Because effective treatment is available, it is important that persons be screened for syphilis on an on-going basis if their sexual behaviors put them at risk for STDs.

Persons who receive syphilis treatment must abstain from sexual contact with new partners until the syphilis sores are completely healed. Persons with syphilis must notify their sex partners so that they also can be tested and receive treatment if necessary.

WILL SYPHILIS RECUR?

Having syphilis once does not protect a person from getting it again. Following successful treatment, people can still be susceptible to re-infection. Only laboratory tests can confirm whether someone has syphilis. Because syphilis sores can be hidden in the vagina, rectum, or mouth, it may not be obvious that a sex partner has syphilis. Talking with a health care provider will help to determine the need to be re-tested for syphilis after treatment has been received.

VAGINITIS

Caused by different germs including yeast and trichomoniasis, vaginitis is an infection of the vagina resulting in itching, burning, vaginal discharge and an odd odor.

WHAT IS BACTERIAL VAGINOSIS?

Bacterial Vaginosis (BV) is the name of a condition in women where the normal balance of bacteria in the vagina is disrupted and replaced by an overgrowth of certain bacteria. It is sometimes accompanied by discharge, odor, pain, itching, or burning.

HOW COMMON IS BACTERIAL VAGINOSIS?

Bacterial Vaginosis (BV) is the most common vaginal infection in women of childbearing age. In the United States, as many as 16 percent of pregnant women have BV.

HOW DO PEOPLE GET BACTERIAL VAGINOSIS?

The cause of BV is not fully understood. BV is associated with an imbalance in the bacteria that are normally found in a woman's vagina. The vagina normally contains mostly "good" bacteria, and fewer "harmful" bacteria. BV develops when there is an increase in harmful bacteria.

Not much is known about how women get BV. There are many unanswered questions about the role that harmful bacteria play in causing BV. Any woman can get BV. However, some activities or behaviors can upset the normal balance of bacteria in the vagina and put women at increased risk including:

- Having a new sex partner or multiple sex

  partners,

- Douching, and

- Using an intrauterine device (IUD) for

contraception.

It is not clear what role sexual activity plays in the development of BV. Women do not get BV from toilet seats, bedding, swimming pools, or from touching objects around them. Women that have never had sexual intercourse are rarely affected.

WHAT ARE THE SIGNS AND SYMPTOMS OF BACTERIAL VAGINOSIS?

Women with BV may have an abnormal vaginal discharge with an unpleasant odor. Some women report a strong fish-like odor, especially after intercourse. Discharge, if present, is usually white or gray; it can be thin. Women with BV may also have burning during urination or itching around the outside of the vagina, or both. Some women with BV report no signs or symptoms at all.

WHAT ARE THE COMPLICATIONS OF BACTERIAL VAGINOSIS?

In most cases, BV causes no complications. But there are some serious risks from BV including:

- Having BV can increase a woman's susceptibility

to HIV infection if she is exposed to the HIV virus.

- Having BV increases the chances that an HIV-infected woman can pass HIV to her sex partner.

- Having BV has been associated with an increase in the development of pelvic inflammatory disease (PID) following surgical procedures such as a hysterectomy or an abortion.

- Having BV while pregnant may put a woman at increased risk for some complications of pregnancy.

- BV can increase a woman's susceptibility to other STDs, such as Chlamydia and gonorrhea.

HOW DOES BACTERIAL VAGINOSIS AFFECT A PREGNANT WOMAN AND HER BABY?

Pregnant women with BV more often have babies who are born premature or with low birth weight (less than 5 pounds).

The bacteria that cause BV can sometimes infect the uterus (womb) and fallopian tubes (tubes that carry eggs from the ovaries to the uterus). This type of infection is called pelvic inflammatory disease (PID). PID can cause infertility or damage the fallopian tubes enough to increase the future risk of ectopic pregnancy and infertility. Ectopic pregnancy is a life-threatening condition in which a fertilized egg grows outside the uterus, usually in a fallopian tube which can rupture.

HOW IS BACTERIAL VAGINOSIS DIAGNOSED?

A health care provider must examine the vagina for signs of BV and perform laboratory tests on a sample of vaginal fluid to look for bacteria associated with BV.

WHAT IS THE TREATMENT FOR BACTERIAL VAGINOSIS?

Although BV will sometimes clear up without treatment, all women with symptoms of BV should be treated to avoid such complications as PID. Male partners generally do not need to be treated. However, BV may spread between female sex partners.

Treatment is especially important for pregnant women. All pregnant women who have ever had a premature delivery or low birth weight baby should be considered for a BV examination, regardless of symptoms, and should be treated if they have BV. All pregnant women who have symptoms of BV should be checked and treated.

Some physicians recommend that all women undergoing a hysterectomy or abortion be treated for BV prior to the procedure, regardless of symptoms, to reduce their risk of developing PID.

BV is treatable with antibiotics prescribed by a health care provider. Two different antibiotics are recommended as treatment for BV: metronidazole or clindamycin. Either can be used with non-pregnant or pregnant women, but the recommended dosages differ. Women with BV who are HIV-positive should receive the same treatment as those who are HIV-negative.

BV can recur after treatment.

About the Author

I was born in a small town in Alabama…nearly the youngest of several siblings. I grew up in a large family and lived in the home with both of my parents throughout my entire childhood years. Family is a very important part of life, which is why I aim high at maintaining a family-oriented environment in our home for my three children.

I lost my dad tragically in a house fire on February 5, 1995. Ten years later I lost my mother on April 10, 2005 after a two year battle with cancer.

It was difficult to lose our mother, being that she was the backbone of the family. She always demonstrated miraculous strength in her life and in raising her children. I can say for the most part that she taught her children how to be strong, and through Christ we were able to handle her death with strength, which is the way she would have wanted us to.

I was inspired by my mother to finish writing this book. Due to health problems, she couldn't do some of the things she wanted to do. I no longer want to linger on the things that have been set before me especially while I am in good health. Occasionally in the past, I have taken life on earth for granted as if it will always be mine. Now, I must press forward to accomplish those things the Lord has set before me for the benefit of others especially our young people.

So, some might ask, "Who is the author?" The answer is a woman of God who gave her life to Christ at the age of thirteen. Challenged with many things in her life, but have compressed those experiences into a message for young adults to apply in their daily lives to achieve and maintain a Christian lifestyle.

Reference:

Http://www.cdc.gov/std, Division of STD
Prevention (DSTDP) Centers for Disease
Control and Prevention

Laird, Charlton/Agnes Michael. Webster's New
World Dictionary and Thesaurus. Cleveland,
Ohio: Wiley Publishing, Inc., 2002

The Scofield Study Bible, King James Version
(KJV). New York, New York: Oxford
University Press, Inc., 2003

Taber's Cyclopedic Medical Dictionary, Edition 20.
2005 by F. A. Davis Company

Wikipedia, The Free Encyclopedia. Version 1.2,
November 2002

National Sexual Assault Online Hotline,
info@rainn.org

CPSIA information can be obtained at www.ICGtesting.com
Printed in the USA
LVOW040142070212

267431LV00001B/2/P

Several years ago the Lord placed on my heart to write a book concerning sexual purity.

He showed me the behavior patterns of children of several grade levels to whom I should be writing. At first it was difficult to decide on my approach of writing, deciding if the contents of my book were to impress or inform. I prayed about my approach of writing, and the Lord revealed to me the importance of simplicity and clarity; so writing by keeping it simple and to the point was the solution. Hopefully, this book will be an informative tool that any child can read and go to the area of his or her spiritual need or needs for answers.

authorHOUSE®

ISBN 978-1-4343-3474-9
90000
9 781434 334749